BACKACHE

Home Treatment and Prevention

Samuel Homola, D.C.

PARKER PUBLISHING COMPANY, INC.   West Nyack, N. Y.

PRINTED IN THE UNITED STATES OF AMERICA

B&P

For my wife, Martha,
and
my mother, Irene

Acknowledgments

The very fine line drawings were
prepared by Bibiana Neal and
Kenneth Faint

Books by the Author

Bonesetting, Chiropractic, and Cultism
Muscle Training for Athletes

A Word to
the Reader

Backache, like the common cold, is one of our most common ailments. But, unlike the mysterious cold infection for which there is no known cause or cure, backache can often be prevented, cured, or alleviated with proper physical care.

About one out of every three people complains of some kind of chronic back trouble, and nearly every one of us, at one time or another, will experience one or more attacks of acute back pain. So even if you are not suffering from back trouble at the present time, the chances are that you will if you do not take the proper steps to prevent it.

If you should develop acute back pain or suffer a serious or painful back injury, or if chronic back trouble should persist or grow worse, you should, of course, see a doctor—and you should follow his advice. But a knowledge of self-help measures will greatly aid your recovery; and by constant observation of certain rules of caution at home, at work, and at play, you can reduce the chances of your back trouble becoming more serious. Furthermore, when you are adequately informed on subjects pertaining to your back and spine, you can avoid many of the everyday irritations that lead to backache.

In any event, most back troubles are of a chronic nature—that is, they cause continuous or recurring discomfort, and how well you get along with this condition will depend largely upon how well you take care of yourself physically. Almost without exception, for example, successful treatment of chronic back trouble, even when under a doctor's care, will hinge upon correct performance of simple procedures that you must follow at home and at work.

According to the U.S. Public Health Service, impairments of the back and spine (excluding paralysis) are the fourth most common cause of varying degrees of chronic disability among the civilian population as a whole. *And among those who are working for a living, impairments of the back and spine are the second most common cause of partial disability or "activity limitation."* [1]

Since most of the disability or discomfort of back trouble can be prevented or alleviated by using simple self-help measures at home, it would be a mistake to ignore your back until you are down and out, and it would be foolish to think that you can take a pill or a single treatment that will quickly erase the structural weaknesses and irritations that have resulted from years of neglect, inactivity, and improper practices. For this reason, the importance of prevention cannot be too strongly stressed. And considering the small amount of time and effort needed to protect your back from strain, you cannot afford not to help yourself when you consider the consequences of disability resulting from back trouble.

As a practitioner specializing in the care of back problems with physical treatment, I have become convinced that *most of our back trouble could be prevented by maintaining good posture, by observing correct lifting techniques, by avoiding emotional stress and strain, and by taking a little regular exercise.* But there are also a multitude of backache-causing irritations in our modern way of living that may not be obvious to you, and you must be told about them if you are to eliminate them.

Thus, with adequate instruction, there is a great deal that you

---

[1] *Chronic Conditions and Activity Limitations,* U.S. Dept. of Health, Education, and Welfare, Washington, D.C., May, 1965.

can do—both in treatment and prevention—to relieve the nagging backache that drags you down at the end of each day, and by continued observation of the simple procedures outlined in this book, you can rid yourself of the slavery of backache, and you can save yourself a lot of time, money, and misery.

Samuel Homola, D.C.

Contents

PART II: HOW TO PREVENT BACKACHE AT HOME AND ON THE JOB

BACKACHE

Home Treatment
and
Prevention

1

What This Book
Can Do for You

As a yearly average, about 28 million people from all walks of life visit doctors' offices in search of relief from backache. Probably a greater number of people annually resort to the use of various non-medical remedies that are even more varied and contradictory than the various treatments employed by some doctors. If you have chronic backache yourself, for example, you may have been visiting doctors and seeking advice on how to relieve your misery. You may have had the confidence-shattering experience of being told by one doctor that you needed back surgery after another doctor had just told you that there was nothing wrong with your back. And you may have learned that some doctors use injections or manipulation, while others recommend traction or corsets. There may even have been some disagreement among the doctors about whether you should use hot packs or cold packs!

If your gardener recommends a "cure," he may swear by bee stings or alfalfa. Your druggist might show you some literature

1

advocating Vitamin C or manganese for "slipped discs," while a health-food enthusiast might recommend bone meal or soya flour. And there are still a few bonesetters around who will pop your neck or gouge the bottom of your foot in treating a sacroiliac strain. I once heard a fisherman recommend a ride on the back of a giant sea turtle for relieving backache.

But in spite of the confusing variety of backache remedies, most of which are worthless, there are many basic home-treatment and prevention techniques that may be used safely by anyone in alleviating or preventing backache, and they have been shown to be scientific, practical, and effective. This book will tell you about these techniques, and it will help you separate fact from fantasy when it comes to taking proper care of your back.

Since most of us already suffer from backache, we do not have to be given a sales talk on the importance of self-help in the care of our affliction. Persons who, so far, have been fortunate enough to escape the pain and humiliating posture of an acute backache need only to take one look at a spraddle-legged back sufferer who is in the throes of agony to appreciate the importance of preventing backache—not to mention the need for adequate treatment.

A FEW SIMPLE HABIT CHANGES OR PRECAUTIONS CAN RELIEVE OR PREVENT BACKACHE

In many cases, a simple alteration in the way we sit, stand, walk, or lift can rescue us from backache troubles.

Consider, for example, the experience of a traveling salesman who had such bad back and leg pains that he had to take strong medication in order to drive from one city to another. And when he arrived at his destination, he sometimes had to have help in getting out of his car. When X-ray examination failed to reveal a cause for his trouble, I questioned him about his sitting posture and his car seat and found that his trouble was apparently due to a prolonged, improper sitting position. All he had to do to get complete relief was to move his car seat up closer to his gas pedal and then suspend a little cushion over the back of his seat for a little additional support in the hollow of his lower back. A simple enough remedy, but worth a "million dollars" to the greatly relieved salesman.

"How to Avoid Motorist's Spine" in Chapter 9 will tell you how to sit properly in your automobile and how to alter your seat for adequate support when necessary.

In another case, a secretary complaining of numbness and tingling in both legs was on the verge of a nervous breakdown from the constant aggravation of her "legs going to sleep." And when she began to experience a weakness in her legs that made it difficult for her to lift her toes up when walking, her nervousness turned to panic. When I examined her one day immediately after she had spent a long day in her office, I noticed two reddened depressions across the back of her thighs just above her knees. It turned out that she had been sitting in an old-style wooden desk chair that was so high and so deep that the edge of the seat was pressing against the back of her thighs just enough to compress important nerves and blood vessels passing down into her legs. She "cured" her trouble simply by switching to a modern secretary's chair that could be adjusted in height to permit a correct sitting posture. Another simple remedy, but another "life saver." (See "How to Sit Correctly for Your Back's Sake" in Chapter 9.)

I can recall one pathetic case of low-back trouble in which a carpenter was in such bad shape that he was in constant agony in performing his work. Because he did not have any source of income other than that he earned in wages, he felt that he had to keep working in order to support his family and to "meet his debts." When he finally did come in for treatment, severe muscle spasm had locked his spine in a grotesquely crooked position, and each step sent a knife-like pain through his lower back. His trouble? One leg was more than an inch shorter than the other, causing his pelvis to tilt down on one side. As a result, a spinal curvature was jamming the joints together on one side of his spine, and every time he took a step his condition was aggravated by a see-sawing pelvis.

The late President Kennedy had the same type of back trouble, and, like the carpenter, he had to wear a lift in one shoe in order to keep his pelvis level and his spine balanced and aligned. Of course, you should not be using a shoe lift without a doctor's advice. But, if you know how to tell whether or not you have a short leg, you might be able to detect the abnormality before it causes trouble—and this can be especially important in the case of children.

I have seen many cases of chronic backache that stemmed directly from bad working postures. I remember one case in particular in which a seamstress in a shirt factory developed such a bad backache in both the upper and lower portions of her spine that she spent her days off (and her savings) going from one doctor to another seeking a cure for what she thought was arthritis. It never occurred to her that the low work bench she crouched over all day was the cause of her trouble. When I called her employer and suggested a change in her working posture, he had the bench elevated and her symptoms gradually disappeared.

Bad posture in any kind of sitting or standing position is, of course, a common cause of backache, both in the joints and in the muscles. Simple postural exercises to realign the joints and to tone up the muscles can relieve such backache, and they can save you from years of misery and chronic disability.

Even a bad sleeping posture can cause backache. Sleeping face down, for example, or simply staying in bed too long, is a common cause of backache. And if a mattress is so soft that the middle of it sags down like a hammock, the spinal joints will be strained in any kind of sleeping posture. I have seen patients spend hundreds of dollars for X-rays, back supports, physical therapy, and office calls in seeking a cure for a nagging backache and then go home each night to sleep on a hollowed-out bed, a broken-down cot, or a deluxe super-soft mattress, even though they had been told many times that a sagging mattress can cause backache. But when backache does occur from inadequate mattress support, it develops so gradually and so insidiously that the cause is not obvious. And the remedy is so simple that it may not be given serious consideration.

"A Firm Mattress Is Important" in Chapter 7 will tell you how to firm up a sagging mattress.

There are an increasing number of backaches that are being caused by improper use of "backache exercises." A 48-year-old sales clerk named Mary G., for example, came in recently complaining of low back pain. "I just don't understand why I have suddenly developed a backache," she said. "I take exercises every Friday night at a beauty school, and the instructor told me they would prevent backache."

"What kind of exercises do you do?" I asked her.

"Well, I do situps, leg raises, and a back-arching exercise . . . and I also do a toe-touching exercise—or I try to."

"What do you mean when you say you 'try to'?"

"I just can't touch my toes, Doctor, no matter how hard I try, and it hurts my back to raise my legs up straight."

When I examined Mary G., I found that her lower spine had been stiffened slightly by a small amount of osteoarthritis. Both her hamstrings and her ankle tendons were so tight that she could not stand on one straight leg (while holding on to a door jamb for balance) and raise the opposite straight leg out in front more than a few feet without feeling a pulling sensation up and down the back of her leg and in her back. And when she tried to go through the same maneuver while lifting her toes up toward her shin, she felt a pain behind her knee.

I also noticed that Mary G. was wearing shoes that had very high heels. When I asked her how long she had been wearing such shoes, she answered: "I've worn them for as long as I can remember."

"What do you wear when you take your exercises?" I asked.

"I wear socks and a sweat suit," she answered, obviously wondering if I knew what I was talking about.

Here is what I told Mary G.: "Mary, you probably need the exercises you are taking, since you have a stiff back as well as tight leg muscles. But you are not doing your exercises properly or often enough. To begin with, your hamstrings and ankle tendons are abnormally short because you have been wearing high-heeled shoes for so long. And when this happens, you can get a backache just by standing around barefooted, and even more so when you exercise without shoes. Of course, you need to stretch those muscles on the back of your legs a little, but you must do it *gradually*. When you do toe-touching exercises forcefully, the terrific pull on the back of your pelvis strains your back. It isn't really necessary to touch your toes. So bend forward slowly, and stop the bending when the pull on the back of your legs begins to get uncomfortable. Wear a pair of shoes that have a little heel on them in order to lessen the tension on the back of your legs while you are standing and exercising. This will also let your back relax a little better. Keep your knees bent during your situps and leg raises so that you can avoid placing too much leverage on your lower spine. And don't arch up as high as you can in your back-arching exercise. Any exercise that places an uncomfortable strain on the back is harmful to the spine. Be guided by how you feel. Try to exercise at least twice a week, on Mondays and Fridays, for example, or every other day if you possibly can. When you exercise only once a week, you don't do the exercises often enough to become accustomed to them."

If you want to take exercise you will have to do it correctly. Chapter 12 will provide detailed instructions in the use of exercises that are designed to strengthen the back without straining the spine. You do not have to become a member of a toe-touching club that creates more backache than it cures.

Remember that lack of exercise is not always the cause of a backache, and exercise itself is only one remedy out of many. But if it is not performed properly it can be a *cause* of backache.

As you will learn in Chapter 10 of this book, incorrect lifting techniques are the most common cause of acute back strain, but you can avoid this type of injury altogether if you know how to lift with your legs instead of with your back. There is also a right way and a wrong way to carry heavy objects. And if you do not push or pull properly, you might suffer a serious back injury, regardless of how strong your muscles are.

Do not wait until you have a backache to make the simple corrections or to observe the simple precautions recommended in this book! You can prevent backache with no trouble at all, but you cannot cure it so easily.

HOME TREATMENT IS SIMPLE BUT EFFECTIVE

When backache or back injury does occur, there are many things that you can do at home to relieve your symptoms and to speed your recovery. Simple moist heat, for example, when properly applied, can provide soothing and relaxing relief for spastic muscles and stiff joints.

There are even safe and simple ways to stretch your spine at home in order to relieve leg pain resulting from a pinched nerve in your spine. "Traction with a Chair," for example, in Chapter 7 tells you how you might be able to relieve low-back pressure simply by draping your legs over the arm of a sofa while you lie on your back on the floor.

I know a business man whose lower vertebrae frequently lock "out of place" to cause muscle spasm that makes it impossible for him to stand erect under his own power—that is, if he does not have his spine stretched. He installed a chinning bar in the doorway of his bedroom and his office for "instant traction." Everytime he feels that peculiar slipping sensation in his spine that begins to tighten up his back muscles, he hangs from the bar and lifts both knees up toward his chest—and *presto*, he feels as good as new!

If you can learn to use such techniques in the care of your own back troubles, you might be able to avoid more drastic forms of treatment, and you can very often prevent the development of the type of backache that takes the joy out of living and the edge off ambition.

Different Types of Backaches Call for Different Remedies

There are many ways to relieve and prevent different types of backache effectively, all of which are discussed in this book—and they may be used by anyone.

You will also learn how bad feet, unpasteurized milk, raw pork, constipation, excessive sweating, exposure to cold, accidents, arthritis, birth defects, structural abnormalities, spinal curvatures, poor diet, overweight, and many other things can cause backache, as well as what you can do about them. You will be told exactly what to do to obtain relief from the backache symptoms that are constantly nagging you to death.

So if you have backache, or if you want to avoid backache, you will find valuable guidance on every page of this book, which has been written especially for *you*. There is even a chapter on how to relax and to relieve or prevent the tension that causes the very common "nervous backache." And at the end of each chapter, there is a summary outlining important information for quick and easy reference. This book tells you everything you will want to know about backache, and in language you can understand.

Exercise Can Be Diagnostic as Well as Preventive

If your back is weak and you need exercise (the five test exercises described at the beginning of Chapter 12 will uncover weak muscles that might cause backache or contribute to back injury), or if your backache is not cleared up simply by avoiding all the stresses and strains that commonly cause backache, there are two chapters at the end of this book describing selected exercises that are designed to strengthen the muscles of your back for better protection of your back and spine. These exercises are simple and easy to do, and they can all be done in the privacy of your bedroom.

Many of the exercises described in Chapter 12 can be used to detect potential causes of back trouble; that is, they can be used as instructed to uncover stiff joints and short muscles and tendons. Try all of the exercises and see if you can do them through a full range of movement. If you find out by doing some of the exercises that you have short hamstrings, tight thigh bands, weak hip flexors, or short ankle tendons, and so on, you can use the same exercises (as instructed) to regain some of your lost flexibility, which will eliminate another potential cause of backache.

If you want to strengthen your body and your back for better back protection in performing heavy work or for participating in strenuous athletics, you will find the barbell exercises in Chapter 13 more effective. And in many cases, you will find that barbell exercises with a small amount of weight are easier and more convenient to do in strengthening certain muscles than free-hand exercises in which you must use your bodyweight.

I have seen many backaches caused by weak, flabby muscles that become inflamed and spastic when placed under abnormal postural stresses. And when such a backache occurs in spongy, deposit-filled muscles, nothing but exercise and improved posture will result in a permanent cure. You can prevent backache that is entirely muscular in origin by taking a little regular exercise *before* backache occurs, and you can prevent loss of your youthful flexibility by starting your exercises *before* you become stiff and tight.

WHY THIS BOOK IS DIVIDED INTO TWO PARTS

Although you should read this book from front to back (regardless of whether your aim is to alleviate or to prevent backache), the material has been divided into two parts for general grouping of treatment and prevention techniques.

Part I, which begins with the next chapter, will tell you about all the things that can go wrong in your back and how to care for them, while Part II, which begins with Chapter 9, will deal primarily with prevention of backache and back injury.

But since prevention should also be a part of treatment, be sure to study both parts of this book if you are really serious about eliminating backache. And keep this book close by for handy reference in handling your back problems from day to day.

Even though backache is one of our most common ailments, you can prevent it in most cases if you have an adequate knowledge of its cause and cure. You do not have to join that army of poor souls who cannot work or play without the constant distraction of a nagging backache.

One expert has said that only about one out of every ten back sufferers shows X-ray evidence of backache-causing *structural defects*. This means that most backaches are probably the result of improper or negligent care for the back.

In any event, when a serious back injury does occur, you can make use of the self-help measures in this book with your doctor's blessings and according to his instructions.

If your doctor has given you a name for your back trouble, but you do not know what it means, you can probably find it described in this book, complete with instructions on what to do about it.

SELF-HELP CAN BE A PLEASURE!

You will enjoy using many of the self-help measures described in this book. The simple massage technique described in Chapter 7, for example, is pure back-rubbing luxury. And the postural exercises described in Chapter 9 should prove to be challenging and entertaining for the whole family.

If you work in a factory or an office, you will find a special set of very simple and welcome rest-break exercises in Chapter 10 that will relieve fatigue and tension, thus benefiting both you and your employer.

If you suffer from backache at the end of each working day, Chapter 8 will tell you how to get some immediate relief from the symptoms caused by various types of work so that you can relax and enjoy your hard-earned rest each night.

There are many important suggestions in this book on how to prevent or alleviate backache, but they are too numerous to mention in an introductory chapter.

You will find all of the information in this book helpful, and in these pages you should find the answer to your particular back problems.

Summary

1. Regardless of how painful or nagging your backache might be, there may be a simple correction that you can make, or a simple treatment that you can use, that will eliminate or relieve your symptoms.
2. But if you want to help yourself, you must be familiar with the various causes of backache, as well as with the various treatments. And that, of course, is the purpose of this book—that is, to help you prevent backache when possible, and then to help you alleviate it when it does occur.

part I

What causes your backache and how to care for it

2

The Many Causes
of Back Trouble

If you have back trouble, you
know that just about *everybody* has back trouble, and all you
have to do to get a lively conversation going in an otherwise
quiet group of people is to ask one long-faced back sufferer how
he is getting along with his infirmity. Chances are, no matter how
terrible, how fantastic, or how excruciating his back trouble may
be, there is always someone in the crowd who has a better story
to tell or whose back trouble is worse. I know one backache victim, for example, who had four unsuccessful spinal operations
for "slipped discs," and who then had to submit to a chordotomy
(cutting a portion of the spinal cord) to relieve the pain in one
of her legs. After the apparently successful cord-cutting operation,
however, she developed a similar pain in the opposite leg!

Not all back trouble is so serious or so difficult to treat. But the
many causes and the varied symptoms of backache make inter-
esting stories, and the talented conversationalist who has polished
up his story about how his back suddenly slipped out of place

and paralyzed him at a crucial moment can be the life of the party.

If you are not a long-time back sufferer, however, you may not be familiar with some of the lingo used by permanent members of the backache club.

GIVING YOUR BACK TROUBLE A NAME

When you hear someone complaining about back trouble, you usually think of the lower back—and most back trouble does occur at the bottom of the spine where stress and strain are the greatest. But the term "back" covers a lot of territory, and in a general way it refers to muscles, bones, joints, ligaments, and tendons in structures that reach all the way from the base of the skull to the tip of the tailbone.

Most doctors refer to disorders involving the joints and ligaments of the vertebral column as "spinal" trouble, while disturbances in muscles, tendons, and other soft tissues around the spine are labeled "back" trouble. In most cases, however, the doctor's diagnosis will also include a term that names the location of the trouble. A "lumbosacral strain," for example, means that the joints and ligaments in a certain portion of the lower back have been strained. A diagnosis of "cervical arthritis" simply means that the bones of the neck are showing signs of arthritis or bone irritation. The very familiar "sacroiliac strain" is easily located by the patient who hobbles along on one leg with his hand braced over the opposite hip.

Low back trouble that does not involve the spine is sometimes called "lumbago," which is a general term that does not imply anything specific (other than pain or soreness in the muscles of the back). Muscular pain between the shoulder blades is often called "dorsal fibromyositis."

Thus, many of the fearsome-sounding names labeling your back troubles are simply generic terms locating and describing your trouble. But if you are afraid of "showing your ignorance" by asking for an explanation of the doctor's diagnosis, you might worry unnecessarily about your condition being more serious than it really is. I had a patient once, for example, who came to me in an obvious state of anxiety because a doctor told him that he had "cervical hypertrophic spondylitis." All he had was a little arthritis in his neck, but the big, long name had stirred up his deepest fears of some terrible disfiguring disease. In another instance, a woman explained that a doctor had examined her neck and told her that she had a "cervical irritation." She wanted to know how a doctor could tell that she had "female trouble" by examining her neck. A farmer complaining of back trouble informed me that he also had "sacolac" (sacroiliac), which he thought was some kind of disease.

There are probably many people who have similar misconceptions about their back trouble simply because they did not ask the doctor for a translation of his medical jargon.

Do not hesitate to ask your doctor what he means if he describes your back trouble in terms that you do not understand. Most doctors are accustomed to using words and phrases that are not in the average layman's vocabulary, and they very often fail to realize that you may have forgotten what you learned in high school biology. Very few dictionaries in homes today include medical terminology, so if you do not ask your doctor about words you do not understand, you may have to make a special and possibly fruitless trip to the library to find out for yourself.

In any event, one of the purposes of this book is to provide you with a working knowledge of your back and spine, in structure as well as in treatment and prevention. And the fact that you are reading this book is a good indication that you will finish it with a practical and comprehensive knowledge of what can happen to your back and what you should do about it.

THINGS THAT CAN GO WRONG IN YOUR BACKBONE

Although man's spine is a mechanical marvel, it is, contrary to popular belief, far from being a perfectly adapted structure; that is, it cannot meet the stress and strain of everyday living without a few things going wrong. The constant pull of gravity upon the vertical and upright spinal column, for example, places a constant strain on the joints and discs of the vertebrae. Unlike the four-legged animal who carries his spine around in a horizontal sling (pity the poor dachshund), the spine of man must support most of his bodyweight when he sits and stands. And in the vertical position, the lower part of the spine is subjected to more weight bearing than the upper part. Furthermore, the transition of the human spine from a horizontal to a vertical position has not yet allowed the vertebral joints to adapt to the stresses of compression. There are also a great many structural defects that are commonly present in the lower spine from birth, and when these are added to the stress and strain of weight bearing it usually means trouble.

Thus, few persons go through life without eventually showing some evidence of disorder or distortion, such as arthritis or spinal curvature. Intervertebral discs (little cushions between the vertebrae) commonly degenerate or herniate under the continuous compression of upright posture. Arthritic spurs sometimes line the vertebral joints with jagged, bony growths, which occasionally press upon nerves and cause severe pain. Structural weakness in what appears to be a normal spine can result in chronic and seemingly incurable back trouble. As a result of causes known and unknown, the spine of a growing child will sometimes sag into a cruel "S"-shape curvature, squeezing the chest and abdominal organs into such a small area that they are unable to function normally (causing death on rare occasions if drastic surgical methods are not employed to halt the progress of the curvature). It is not uncommon for X-ray photographs of the spine to reveal extra vertebrae or an excessive number of ribs; for example, there may be six lumbar vertebrae (in the lower portion of the spine) instead of five, or there may be a "cervical rib" in the neck just above the normal first rib.

Malformations of every conceivable type can occur in any portion of the spinal column, any one of which can cause varying amounts of discomfort or pain. Many of these disorders will be discussed in other chapters of this book.

EMPLOYMENT AS A CAUSE OF "RETIREMENT BACKACHE"

We all know that accidents can cause back trouble, and we will learn how to avoid these accidents in other portions of this book; but few people realize that a back injury today can cause back trouble 10 years from now. A policeman who is thrown somersaulting from his motorcycle in a collision, for example, may complain of "slipped disc" or arthritis many years after the accident. A painter who had to jump from a falling ladder may begin to "feel" his back many years after he "got over" the initial back sprain.

Persons who do the type of work that subjects the spinal joints

and discs to continuous jarring, compression, or awkward postures may begin to experience back trouble after retirement, even
though they "never missed a day's work in 20 years on the job."
A coal miner, a heavy equipment operator, a circus acrobat, a
paratrooper, or a construction worker, for example, commonly
complains of back trouble after retirement. In time to come, I
would imagine that astronauts who repeatedly experience ac-
celeration and deceleration in cramped sitting positions would
also be candidates for "retirement backache."

There is, of course, a simple and logical explanation for the
delayed occurrence of chronic back trouble resulting from occu-
pation or employment. It is well known among doctors that
when the joints or discs are subjected to continuous strain or to
repeated minor injuries—not to mention one or more severe injuries—certain changes take place over the joint surfaces or in
the disc fibers as time goes by. The fibers of a disc, for example,
that has been injured in a fall or in stooped working postures,
may begin to degenerate, so that the disc either ruptures at a
later date or just deteriorates until it practically disappears from
between the vertebrae. Joint surfaces that are injured in a bad
accident or repeatedly banged together by the jarring of a daily
tractor ride over rough terrain will frequently undergo a slow
arthritic reaction that results in bone and calcium formation
around the injured joints and ligaments. It may be several years
before the formations are large enough to cause trouble.

*Thus, what you are doing today has a great deal to do with
how your back will fare in the years to come.* So if you have a
choice, try to avoid work in which strains, injuries, accidents,
or repeated jarring might injure your spine. As far as I know,
very few companies offer compensation for "retirement backache" that results from past employment, since it may be difficult
or impossible to prove that employment was the cause of the
disability.

I have seen a number of patients who developed back trouble
several years after an accident or an injury. A former air force
man, for example, began to experience back pain from a "loose"
vertebra in his spine (see "Spondylolisthesis—The Wandering
Vertebra" in Chapter 4) ten years after he fell from an airplane
and struck his lower back on a ladder. A war-time Navy Seabee

had to have a hip joint repaired with a steel ball and socket when the bone in his hip began to crumble like chalk. He was suffering from "avascular necrosis," which means that the affected bone was dying from lack of adequate blood circulation—and it was the result of an injury he had suffered 15 years ago when a large beam struck him on the hip. A civil service worker began to experience severe, localized symptoms of arthritis and disc degeneration in his neck several years after he had injured his neck in a near-fatal accident while he was on the job. But because the symptoms did not develop within two years after his apparent recovery from the accident, his workmen's compensation insurance did not cover his disability.

WHAT PERSISTENT BACK PAIN CAN MEAN

Fortunately, serious and deadly bone diseases and infections that occur in the spine are rarely a cause of back pain, but it is important that an effort be made to detect such disorders as soon as possible. Always see your family physician when acute back pain develops, but if the pain should get worse after one week of treatment, or if it does not improve after two weeks of treatment, your back should be examined by an orthopedic or bone specialist.

Many infectious and malignant conditions causing back pain can be cured in their early stages, but if they should be allowed to progress under a careless diagnosis of lumbago, nervous tension, or occupational strain, the consequences can be fatal. For this reason, *any unlabeled or persistent back pain should be examined by an orthopedic specialist and a radiologist (X-ray specialist) to eliminate possible bone disease.* If examination fails to reveal a cause for the pain, and the family physician cannot find an organic disturbance that might be referring pain into the structures of the back (see "Back Trouble That Isn't Back Trouble" in Chapter 3), the examinations should be repeated periodically until the cause of the pain is discovered. Some bone diseases, for example, cause back pain for several weeks before they become apparent on X-ray examination.

I knew one middle-aged man who developed back and leg pain for which no apparent cause could be found but which resembled the symptoms of a "slipped disc." His family physician prescribed medication and suggested that he see an orthopedic specialist if the pain persisted. For some reason, however, the man did not seek further examination or treatment until the pain became unbearable (in spite of the continued use of drugs!). When he finally did check into a large clinic for treatment, doctors found that he had a malignant bone disease that was eating away the bone in the bottom of his spine.

Thus, although backache is rarely caused by serious bone disease, back pain should never be ignored for very long simply because you have a constant supply of pain pills.

Any sudden backache or back pain that is accompanied by fever, headache, and other symptoms of illness should be brought to the attention of your family physician immediately. There are a large number of minor and serious infectious diseases that cause backache. In fact, there is hardly a systemic infection of any kind that does not result in some degree of backache. Every home should have a thermometer for routine checking of the body temperature when pain or illness occurs.

Not long ago, a 25-year-old mechanic walked into my office complaining of backache. He told me that he had hurt his back while installing a motor in an old car. When a case history and a physical examination failed to point to a possible back injury, I took his temperature and found that it was 102 degrees Fahrenheit. Yet, his only complaint was backache! X-ray examination revealed that he had a type of "virus pneumonia," so he was referred to a nearby medical practitioner for treatment.

Since any kind of backache that is accompanied by fever usually has an infectious origin, you should go first to your family doctor or to a general medical practitioner rather than to an orthopedic specialist or a chiropractor if use of a thermometer at home reveals an abnormally high temperature.

DIAGNOSIS IS IMPORTANT

Correct treatment of any acute backache or back pain will, of course, depend first upon getting a correct diagnosis. When a backache is caused by an infection, for example, it is the infection and not the back that must be treated. And if there is a spinal disorder requiring spinal manipulation, no amount of heat, massage, or exercise will do the job. On the other hand, if you have chronic backache resulting from weak muscles, poor posture, bad lifting habits, dietary indiscretions, and other self-imposed factors, treatment is largely your responsibility after a diagnosis has been made.

Of course, you should always make an effort to correct any potential cause of backache, whether you think it is causing your backache or not; and you should observe such precautions as a matter of prevention, even if you do not have backache. But do not try to diagnose your own trouble if you have a persistent or severe backache. Let your doctor find out what is wrong with your back and then follow his instructions.

I had a patient once who came in with great reluctance for treatment. And since he had already compared his symptoms with those of a neighbor who had a simple but aggravating case of osteoarthritis, he informed me that all he needed was a little diathermy (heat). When I took his case history and found that there was reason to suspect the presence of spinal gout (see "The Big-Toe Pain in Your Back" in Chapter 6), I suggested that he try eliminating two of his favorite foods—wine and poultry—from his diet, since they might have been a source of a form of acid that was causing "gouty arthritis" or joint inflammation. The disgruntled patient, who had already made up his mind about what he thought his trouble was, stalked out of my office and went from doctor to doctor until he found one who told him exactly what he wanted to hear. The last time I saw him, he was hobbling around on crutches, and I suspected from the bright red color of his nose and his joints that he was still drinking wine instead of water.

COMMON CAUSES OF BACKACHE

Actually, fatal, crippling, or serious conditions causing backache or back pain are relatively rare. For the most part, the most common causes of backache can be eliminated by exercising good posture, by maintaining well-toned muscles, by lifting properly, by avoiding physical and emotional stress and strain, and by observing the rules of healthy living.

Many back injuries occur because the muscles are not strong enough to prevent tearing or "pulling" of muscle fibers during sudden or heavy exertion in unaccustomed activities, or because the muscles and tendons are not tight enough to prevent the wrenching of a spinal joint during an awkward movement. Thick and well-toned muscles are taut and elastic, thus providing a high degree of protection for the joints and their ligaments. Once the muscles become small, spongy, and lax, however, the integrity of the joint then depends largely upon overworked and more easily strained ligaments, especially when posture is bad.

As you will learn in Chapter 9, poor posture alone is a major cause of backache. If you sit and stand improperly, you will have backache, no matter how much exercise you take. I knew a struggling writer who had chronic backache and who took a course of popular exercises that were designed to strengthen the back and restore flexibility to relieve backache. The exercises were, of course, good, and he probably needed them; but since weak muscles were not causing his backache, the exercises did not eliminate his backache. After several weeks of regular exercise, he dropped in for a consultation and we reviewed the possible causes of his type of backache. It turned out that he did a great deal of his writing in a rocking chair with his notebook placed on the arm of the chair or on the knee of a crossed-over leg. As a result, he had developed the habit of tilting his pelvis so that most of his bodyweight was supported on one buttock when he sat down, and this caused a type of functional curvature of his spine that was evident only in a sitting position. I instructed him in proper sitting postures and suggested that he write on the kitchen table or buy a desk that he could brace his elbows on and slip his legs under. After a little difficulty in becoming accustomed to the change in his habitual writing posture, he got rid of his backache and increased his writing output.

As you will learn in other portions of this book, various unavoidable working postures are a common cause of backache, and sometimes nothing but a change in jobs will relieve such a backache. A good example of this was presented to me recently when a young, muscular plumber came in complaining of back pain between his shoulder blades. He had all the symptoms of spinal arthritis, but X-ray examination was negative. Since he was an apprentice for a very busy plumbing firm, he had been assigned the task of crawling up under houses to dig trenches and hookup plumbing. "That's the cause of your trouble," I told him. "The awkward and tiring postures you must assume under those houses is causing an arthritic-like joint inflammation. And you'll probably continue to experience it as long as you do that kind of work."

"I can't quit my job, Doctor," the plumber said, "and they won't let me skip that phase of my job training."

So we tried everything—special exercises, manipulation, traction, the works. And he followed the self-help procedures described under "The Backache of Over-Exertion" in Chapter 8. With his cooperation, we managed to keep his symptoms relieved enough to permit continued working, but he did not completely get rid of his backache until he "graduated" to the status of a full-fledged plumber who could assign the under-house "dirty work" to a helper.

Nowadays, when I ask a patient about his back, I also ask him about his job.

Tall people especially are subject to postural backache. And when they try to hide their height by slumping, backache is inevitable.

Correct Lifting Techniques Are Especially Important!

Even when the muscles are strong and well-developed and the posture is good, joint strain can occur rather easily in awkward or improper lifting techniques. A professional weightlifter, for example, can lift a tremendous amount of weight overhead by using scientific lifting technique in which he has control over the use of his muscles, and he can do it without strain or injury. But if he should attempt to lift a lighter object in an awkward position, as in trying to lift a large bag of groceries out of the back seat of a car, he might place a considerable amount of leverage on his spine at a moment when his muscles are relaxed or off guard, thus straining his back.

Back strain can also occur rather easily when there is an unexpected interruption of movement in walking or lifting. If you are walking along and you stumble over a rug or some other object, for example, the sudden jerk of your muscles in recovering your balance can strain muscles, joints, and ligaments. The same thing can happen if you step into a hole or off a curb unexpectedly. If you are told to lift an object from the floor, and it is a great deal heavier than you expected it to be, you might suffer a serious strain if you attempted the lift without first testing the actual weight of the object.

Thus, no matter how strong you are, you should lift in guarded, controlled movements in which there is as little leverage as possible on your spine, or you might suffer a painful back injury that is more serious than the simple backache of bad posture. You will get all the details of how to lift correctly in Chapter 10, along with specific instructions on how to avoid back-crippling accidents at home and on the job.

A STATE OF MIND MAY BE INVOLVED IN BACKACHE

As you are beginning to see, backache can be a complicated subject, and sometimes there is more involved than just muscles, bones, and ligaments. Anytime a patient complains of a backache that does not have an obvious mechanical cause, for example, doctors have learned that there may even be mental or emotional factors involved. So do not feel insulted if a doctor should ask you about your emotional problems as well as about your job and your habits in trying to uncover the cause of your backache.

Chapter 11 will tell you how your nerves can cause simple backache and what you can do about it yourself. But let me tell you about a case of nervous backache that provided a clue to an impending nervous breakdown.

A Case of Mental Strain Causing Backache

A 33-year-old married woman complaining of backache described her pain as "unbearable." Yet, she slept soundly at night and was so "exhausted" that she always overslept in the mornings. She had "no energy" to do her housework, and the children were "impossible to handle."

"This backache is getting me down," she said. "I cry all day, and everything is beginning to get on my nerves."

When physical and X-ray examination did not reveal anything wrong with her back, I asked her if she was under any kind of nervous or emotional strain, and she told me a very emotional story about how miserable she was and how "inconsiderate and unfaithful" her alcoholic husband was. Neither the husband nor the wife would agree to seek specialized care, however, and both became hopelessly entangled in their problems—he in his alcoholism and extra-marital affairs and she in her emotional illness.

The poor woman's backache grew worse, and she began to develop many other distressing symptoms. She got a cinder in her eye and thought she was going blind. Her menstruation was a little heavier than usual and she thought she was bleeding to death. She felt sure that the stomach gas pains she had were being caused by cancer. Then one day her anxiety overwhelmed her and she began screaming hysterically. Something snapped, and her mind withdrew into a quiet little corner where she could be alone and unbothered.

Fortunately, this story has a happy ending. The woman recovered under proper psychiatric care, and the husband, who realized for the first time what he was doing to his wife, underwent a cure for his alcoholism. The last time I saw them, they were husband and wife again, and the happy, radiant woman no longer had a backache.

Of course, your chances of having a nervous breakdown are small, but the point is that if you or any member of your family should experience such severe emotional problems as those related in the case above, make sure that you get proper counseling. Do not let your back be a scapegoat. If personal and family problems are not recognized for what they are and corrected before they get out of hand, your nervous backache could lead to more serious trouble.

Don't Wait Until It's Too Late!

Although most chronic back disorders could be prevented by proper attention to various prophylactic measures (all of which will be discussed in detail throughout this book), it seems, strangely enough, to be very much a part of human nature for "healthy" persons to procrastinate in adopting a program of preventive measures. Yet, many people will rush to the office of a doctor, when pain occurs, seeking a sudden and complete cure for a condition that has been years in the making and that is (in the spine, at least) sometimes incurable—as far as complete recovery goes—because of irreversible structural or bony changes. Many years of habitually bad posture, for example, causing an extreme exaggeration of the normal curves of the spine, can cause a wedge-shaped deformity in vertebrae that have been molded under abnormal stresses, making it impossible to stand perfectly straight. And repeated injury to joints and ligaments can result in loose, arthritic, and unstable joints that cause constant or recurring backache. You cannot get away with abusing your back and spine and then waiting until you have a backache to make the necessary corrections.

The General Pattern of Chronic Backache

Most of the foundation for chronic back trouble is probably laid down before the individual reaches 25 years of age; that is, of course, in disturbances that are not related to injury or disease. Structural weaknesses and congenital (birth) defects in the spine almost always cause trouble when the muscles grow weak from inactivity or old age. Thus, many young people who develop spinal distortions through bad posture may not begin to feel the effects of their bad habits until the changes of age take place; that is, when the discs begin to get thin and a sagging, unbalanced spine begins to grind arthritic formations together. Obviously, good posture during youth is the first important approach to good spinal health, but the older we become—good posture or not—the more important it becomes to take a little regular exercise.

As a general rule, persons who neglect the basic rules of caring for their back and spine in their formative years have no one but themselves to blame when structural weaknesses appear that could have been prevented, but children are sometimes forced to assume responsibility for their own care with severe physical handicaps that have been allowed to develop by negligent and thoughtless parents who fail to fulfill their parental duties in molding the habits of their children. If you have children, you should stress the importance of good posture, exercise, and other body-strengthening measures that will aid in the physical development of *every* member of the family.

Once developed, good habits are not thought of as being inconvenient or "too much trouble." Keep this in mind as you read and follow the various recommendations offered in this book for preventing and overcoming back trouble. A little inconvenience directed toward acquiring a habit of prevention is priceless when compared with chronic disability later. So whether you have a backache or not, you should begin *now* to exercise prevention at home and on the job.

As you learned in Chapter 1, most backaches are caused by stresses and strains that can be removed immediately by making a few simple changes in the way you work, play, and rest. And if you are well informed about the various causes of backache —and you will be if you read this book—you can eliminate many harmful stresses before they affect *your* back.

Summary

1. Remember that there is a difference between backache and acute back pain. If you have chronic backache, there is a great deal that you can do to help yourself, and you can prevent many types of back pain and backache by observing the rules of back care outlined in this book. But if your back trouble should persist, or if you should suddenly develop an acute backache or back pain, you should be examined by a doctor, especially when the symptoms are accompanied by fever and other symptoms of illness.

2. When backache of undetermined origin is accompanied by great anxiety or emotional outbursts, the cause of the backache may have a mental rather than a physical origin. So do not hesitate to tell your doctor about your personal problems if he should ask you about them.

3. The type of work you do and the way you live, as well as the strains and injuries you suffer, may lay the groundwork for back trouble in the years to come. For this reason, you should begin *now* to protect your spine from abnormal stresses and strains—and you can do this by maintaining good posture during work, play, sleeping, sitting, and standing; by lifting correctly; by avoiding accidents; by keeping your muscles strong; and by maintaining a tranquil mind. All of these preventive measures will be thoroughly covered in Part II of this book.

4. If you already have a backache, you will find many simple self-help and preventive suggestions in the chapters to follow.

5. Do not be discouraged just because you have had a backache for a long time. Experience has shown that most
   backaches can be alleviated when the cause is known.
   So if you will follow the instructions offered in this book,
   you have every reason to be optimistic about making a
   full recovery.

3

What You Should Know
About Your Back
and Spine

One of the first steps to be taken in beginning a program of self-help measures that are designed to prevent or relieve backache is to acquire a basic knowledge of the structures of the back and spine and how they work. If you have some idea of what the normal spine should look like, and if you are familiar with the function of the back muscles in putting the spine into motion, you will be able to lift, exercise, and stand more efficiently—and you will be able to alter your activities to your best advantage when necessary. An automobile driver or an airplane pilot, for example, must have some knowledge of how his machine works if he is to know what to do when something goes wrong, and the same holds true for your body, especially your back. Of course, your body has many built-in warning signals that may give you some indication of when to lie down, when to stand up, and when to rest; but, as in operating a machine, there are certain techniques and procedures that must be used and observed in correcting or preventing a "breakdown" of the supporting structures in your back, and these must be learned.

One of the best examples I know of that stresses the need for a knowledge of what a normal back and spine should look like is presented daily in doctors' offices where parents learn, for the first time, that their teenage son or daughter has a bad spinal curvature that should have been attended to several years earlier. Because of the average parent's inability to visualize the structures of the spine, many correctable disorders of the spine are overlooked as being poor posture or birth deformity. A child with one leg shorter than the other, for example, may be accused of having "poor character" for not standing "straight" like his playmates; or the difference in the size of the breasts of a young girl whose spine is twisted may be shrugged off as an unfortunate "female deformity."

There are many cases where a knowledge of the back's architecture can be helpful in preventing or relieving pain. It is good to know, for example, how low back trouble can cause leg pain, even when you do not feel any pain in your back. When you understand how this can happen, you can better heed nature's signals by assuming corrective postures. Furthermore, if you know how your muscles support your back, you can relieve fatigue, strain, and muscle spasm by correcting daily job stresses in a "tailor-made" manner.

THE IMPORTANCE OF KNOWING THE MECHANICS OF YOUR BACK

Thomas Jefferson once wrote that "Health is no more than learning." And this is true in the beginning, especially when it comes to something as complicated as your back and spine. So before you begin considering actual measures of treatment and prevention, you should know something about the mechanics of your "back."

YOUR COMPLICATED BACKBONE

If you stripped all the muscles away from the spinal column, you would have a semi-rigid structure resembling a crooked banana stalk. The ligaments binding the individual vertebrae together would be so thick and numerous that you would barely be able to distinguish one vertebra from another, and most of the complex spinal joints would be hidden from view.

Actually, there are 26 vertebrae in the spine, and, counting the rib joints of the vertebrae but excluding the "disc joints," there are about 97 joints in the spine itself. One authority has said that if you include all the attachments of the skull, the ribs, and the pelvis where they hook up to the vertebral column, there are about 135 real and false joints (in our backbone) that have joint sacs (called "synovial sacs" by your doctor) where "joint trouble" may develop.

So you can see that movement of the spinal column by even more complex muscle action is a doubly complex process.

How Your Spine Is Constructed from Top to Bottom

The spine itself is divided into 5 main sections: cervical, dorsal, lumbar, sacral, and coccygeal.

The Cervical or Neck Spine

The cervical or neck portion of the spine is made up of seven vertebrae. Because it supports the head, it must be able to swivel, bend, rotate, and go through a variety of movements in order to direct the senses of sight, hearing, smell, and taste effectively. If you have ever had a "stiff neck," or if you have ever seen anyone who had a fused or badly injured neck, you can readily appreciate the function and the importance of cervical flexibility.

The first vertebra of the neck is called the "atlas," and it is so named because of its function in supporting the skull; that is, it was named after Atlas, the mythical Greek Titan whose job it was to support the heavens on his shoulders.

The atlas sits on the "axis," the second vertebra of the neck, where it rotates about a vertical, dowel-like projection of bone.

The rest of the cervical vertebrae have no peculiar distinguishing characteristics (although each vertebra is slightly different from the others), so they are simply numbered from 3 to 7. However, the seventh cervical vertebra at the bottom of the neck has a long bony process that projects backward far enough to cause a

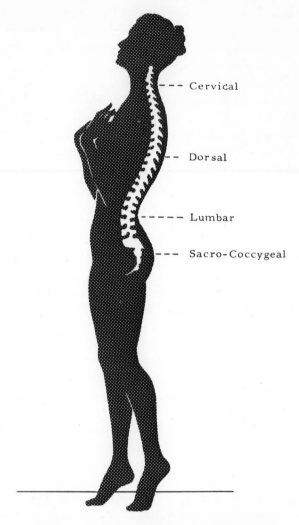

Cervical

Dorsal

Lumbar

Sacro-Coccygeal

Figure 1:   Normal curves of the spine

large, visible "bump" (on the back of the neck where the neck joins the shoulders) when the head is tilted down. Very often, persons who are having neck trouble for the first time will discover this bump and then worry about it being some kind of growth. It may be more prominent in some than in others, but it is normal. Doctors call it the "vertebral prominens." Tilt your head down and feel this bump, and then feel it in the same way in the neck of a couple of your friends.

All of the vertebrae of the spine except the atlas have a finger-like process of bone that projects backward toward the skin (spinous process), and they are all visible as bony bumps up and down the center of the back. Of course, these bumps are more visible in thin persons than in heavy persons, and they may not be visible at all in very fat persons. Just the other day, an 80-year-old woman who had lost a great deal of weight asked me if the bumps up and down her spine—which were becoming increasingly prominent as she lost weight—were arthritic growths.

Each vertebra also has bony "transverse processes" which project out on each side for the attachment of muscles. These processes are not visible, but they can be felt on each side of the neck in thin persons. In fact, more than one anxious patient has visited a doctor to inquire about these "lumps" in his neck.

When the neck is normal, the cervical spine makes up about one-fifth of the total length of the spinal column, and its curve bends toward the front of the body. Occasionally, however, there may be an improper number of cervical vertebrae or there may be some kind of deformity that will stiffen the neck and make it appear abnormally short (Klippel-Feil deformity) or long, and the normal curve may straighten out or reverse itself (visible only on X-ray examination). In fact, people who have any kind of neck trouble will very often have a reversed cervical curve, which may result in tension headaches, "cricks," or sore neck muscles. Corrective exercise can improve this condition, however, and I have described a neck exercise for this purpose in Chapter 12. This exercise can be done safely by anyone for corrective or preventive purposes.

The Dorsal or Upper Spine

The dorsal or thoracic portion of the spine is composed of 12 vertebrae which have 24 spinal joints and 24 rib joints. (If you count the rib joints at the transverse processes and on the vertebrae, there are 84 joints in the dorsal spine! This little bit of worthless information will give you some idea of how complex your spine really is.)

Unlike the neck, the dorsal spine is somewhat limited in its movements because of the attachment of the ribs to the vertebrae, and the column of bones curves toward the back rather than toward the front as the cervical spine does. The alternating curves of the spine make the vertebral column more flexible and about 16 times stronger than if it were straight, however, and they aid in absorbing the shocks placed on the spine when it is in an erect position. Just imagine what a rough ride your brain would get if your skull were supported by a straight, rigid spine.

The curves of the spine also mold themselves to the organs of the body in order to protect them and to enhance their function. With the dorsal spine curving backward, for example, and the ribs flaring out in front, there is room for the lungs to expand and the heart to function. When the dorsal curve sags from poor posture or from weak muscles, poor health may result, in addition to many aches and pains in the muscles, joints, and ligaments.

The normal curves of the spine are, of course, visible only when viewing the body from the side. And when the dorsal curve is greatly exaggerated, it causes a hump-back type of posture in which the head is thrust forward, which in turn increases the normal curve of the neck. Thus, persons who have such bad posture that the head is centered in front of the mid-line of the body almost always have neck trouble—in addition to back trouble—from constant tension on the neck muscles and from a jamming together of the joints, which can cause headache or arm pain from nerve irritation. All of this can be prevented, however, simply by taking the postural exercises outlined in Chapter 9.

When the body is viewed from the front or the back, the spine should appear to be nearly straight. Very few people have a perfectly straight spine, however, and *Gray's Anatomy* now tells us that it is normal for the dorsal spine to curve a little toward the arm we use most. A right-handed person, for example, might have a slight right dorsal curve, while a left-handed person might have a little curve to the left—provided, of course, there are no structural defects in the spine causing an abnormal curvature.

In any event, a perfectly straight spine (in viewing it from the back on X-ray examination) is not very common. But if you do not avoid an exaggeration of the normal curves of your spine by maintaining good posture and by taking a little regular exercise, you may be headed for trouble. Gravity is a relentless foe of the upright spinal column, so you will have to make a conscious and consistent effort to keep it erect.

The Lumbar or Lower Spine

The lumbar or low-back section of the spine is composed of five vertebrae, and its curve is directed toward the front of the body. When the normal lumbar curve is exaggerated, it results in the sway-back type of posture that is so familiar to all of us.

As you will find out by reading the rest of this book, most of our back trouble occurs in the lumbar portion of our spine, for two reasons: (1) because the lumbar spine supports most of the body weight, and (2) because there are a greater number of bony abnormalities in the lumbar vertebrae than anywhere else in the spine. It is not at all uncommon, for example, to find six lumbar vertebrae instead of five; and occasionally there will be only four.

Like the cervical spine, the lumbar spine will sometimes flatten out or reverse itself (curve backward) when something goes wrong, although the sway-back deformity is most common.

Needless to say, exercise and good posture are very important in keeping the low back strong, flexible, and balanced in order to protect the joints, discs, ligaments, and nerves. Improper lifting techniques, however, are the most common cause of acute back strain, so the how-to-lift instructions in Chapter 10 will be a valuable part of your back-care program.

The Sacral or Pelvic Spine

The sacral portion of the spine is formed by the sacrum, a single wedge-shaped bone that is lodged between the two pelvic bones. Unlike the cervical, dorsal, and lumbar portions of the spine, there is no voluntary movement in the sacral spine itself, since the sacrum and the pelvis must move as a unit. There are a number of muscles attaching to the sacrum, but only to anchor for the movement of other joints.

In any event, the sacrum is wedged down and locked between the pelvic bones by irregular joint surfaces that are molded to each other and bound together by very strong and dense ligaments. No movement at all is possible in an up-and-down direction, but under heavy stress it is possible for a pelvic bone to rotate on the sacrum, resulting in a very painful sacroiliac strain.

Since most sacroiliac strains are caused by improper lifting, special care should be taken to avoid lifting techniques that place leverage or twisting strains on the lower back. (The lifting techniques described in Chapter 10 are designed to provide maximum protection for the sacroiliac joints.)

Although the sacrum is considered to be only one vertebra, it is actually made up of five segments that fuse together at about 25 years of age.

The sacral spine curves backward, and is largely responsible for the curve of the buttocks. I have seen a number of patients with prominent sacral curves who thought they were sway-backed.

The Coccyx or "Tail-Bone" Spine

The coccyx or "tail bone" is a small segmented bone attached to the bottom of the sacrum. Although it has no obvious function other than to serve as an attachment site for certain pelvic muscles, it is not infrequently the site of discomfort or pain, especially when it is subjected to prolonged pressure—as in improper sitting —or direct blows. You should never kick anyone from behind, and you should never pull the chair out from under someone as a prank. Once the coccyx is injured or strained, it can cause chronic, painful symptoms that are difficult to cure.

If your child has a prominent tail bone—that is, if it protrudes like a small tail—let an orthopedic surgeon remove it. Medical records indicate that tail bones as long as three inches have been seen in newborn babies.

There are four segments in the normal coccyx, but they fuse together at about the age of 25 or 30. If you should read somewhere that the spine has 33 vertebrae, remember that this includes the segments of both the sacrum and the coccyx.

Although we can get along without our lowly tail bone, the Jews, Christians, and Mohammedans once believed that this "indestructible" little bone was the "resurrection bone" from which life would once again reappear.

The coccyx, of course, is a very small bone, and it fits into the curve of the sacrum.

Thus, from the top of your spine to the bottom, there are four major curves: a cervical curve to the front, a dorsal curve to the back, a lumbar curve to the front, and a sacro-coccygeal curve to the back.

In addition to providing protection for the body's organs, these curves account for much of the beauty and shape of the body, and they keep the body properly centered and balanced for the dynamic posture we all need to look good and to show "get up and go." Persons with bad posture are not only unattractive physically, but very often lack the self-confidence and the vigor needed to really get ahead in this world.

The Lumbosacral Joints—The Crossroads of Backache

The lumbosacral joints of the spine are formed where the lumbar spine and the sacral spine come together. Because of weight-bearing defects that are commonly present in these joints, plus the fact that the movable fifth lumbar vertebra sits on a rigid, immovable sacrum, most low-back aches and pains occur at the bottom of the lumbar spine.

It used to be the fashion to say that one had a "sacroiliac strain" when he had a back pain, but most of the time the trouble was actually in the lumbosacral joints.

If you have been around for a while, you might remember this little ditty that was so popular back in the "sacroiliac days":

"My spine's out of whack. . . . There's a great big crack . . . in the back . . . of my sacroiliac."

Nowadays, everyone complains of having a "slipped disc," but most of the trouble is still in the lumbosacral joints.

In any event, all of the common causes of backache can cause lumbosacral strain. I do a great deal of writing, and I frequently experience mild symptoms of low back strain from prolonged sitting. Chapter 4 will tell you how you commonly injure the joints of your spine.

THE INTERVERTEBRAL DISCS—YOUR SPINE'S "BUILT-IN" SHOCK ABSORBERS

In addition to the cushioning effect of the normal spinal curves, there are small cartilage-like cushions separating the individual vertebrae. These are called "intervertebral discs," and they are the culprits in the so-called "slipped disc" injuries.

There are no discs between the skull and the atlas, between the atlas and the axis, or between the sacrum and the coccyx; so there are only 23 discs for 26 vertebrae.

In the erect posture assumed by man, the intervertebral discs support most of the weight placed on the spine, and they serve as "ligaments" to bind the vertebrae together. The gristle-like discs are flexible enough to permit the spine to bend, and they are filled with a jelly-like substance that cushions the vertebrae.

When a disc is weak, the semi-liquid material in the center of the disc bulges out from between the vertebrae to resemble a weak spot on an inflated inner tube. When a disc ruptures, however, the soft center of the disc may seep out and cause so much trouble that it may have to be removed surgically.

In any event, when a disc fails to keep the vertebrae adequately separated and cushioned, the spinal joints may jam against each other to cause various kinds of joint pain. Normally, the spinal joints do not support any weight at all, and they serve only to guide and protect the movement of the vertebrae. But when a disc ruptures or degenerates, the joints must assume some of the job of supporting the bodyweight, and this means trouble, especially if there are other disturbances in the joints (such as bone abnormality or arthritis).

Of course, as we grow older, the discs naturally become thinner from aging, dehydration, and wear and tear. This is why old people complain of "growing shorter" along with chronic backache as they grow older. And if the normal curves of the spine sag as the muscles become weaker from lack of exercise, there may be a pronounced loss of height and backache may be greatly aggravated. Thus, if you do not develop good posture and keep your back muscles strong as you grow older, you may experience a great deal of back trouble when age begins to ravage the cushions between your vertebrae. And if you do not lift correctly, regardless of how young you might be, you may rupture a disc with excessive pressures.

When the discs are normal and healthy, they form approximately one-fourth of the total length of the spinal column. After a long day of standing and sitting, the thickness of the discs will decrease a little from the compression placed on them by the weight of the body, but when we go to bed at night we regain the height we lost during the day, which is sometimes as much as three-quarters of an inch.

There are some people who claim that their spine can be stretched several inches when placed under traction, but most of this increase in length is simply a straightening out of the normal curves of the spine. It is possible, of course, to increase height temporarily by repeated stretching of the spine, and more than one job applicant has walked directly from a traction table to an examining room when a slight increase in height was needed to meet physical requirements.

In any event, since just about everything we do during the day places compression strain on the spine and its discs, it might be a good idea to lie down occasionally during the day or to hang from a bar for a few moments in order to let the discs expand. This would also relieve tension on the joints and muscles, and it would permit separation of the joints enough for the joint fluids to lubricate the joint surfaces.

How Your Spine Protects Your Nerves

In addition to serving as a central support for all of the structures of the body, the spinal column also serves as a lifeline between the body and the brain. On the back of each vertebra, for example, there is a bony ring (on a horizontal plane) which, in formation with the rings of all the other vertebrae, forms a spinal canal for passage and protection of the spinal cord (which is literally an extension of the brain). The spinal canal itself is filled with a long, fluid-filled sac that houses and protects the spinal cord; and the normal curves of the vertebral column, along with 26 movable segments, permit the spine to bend and turn without kinking the spinal cord.

The individual nerve trunks branching out from the spinal cord to supply various parts of the body pass through bony openings formed by a notch on the vertebra above and the vertebra below, which come together to form an intervertebral foramen. With one exception (at the lumbosacral joint where the opening fits snugly about the nerve), these openings are much larger than the nerves which pass through them, and they are padded with fatty tissue and blood vessels to prevent bony irritation or pressure from movement of the vertebrae. Thus, the spinal nerves are seldom pressed upon or pinched unless some kind of disorder—such as arthritis, a "slipped disc," a tumor, or an injury—is present.

Bad posture, however, can result in irritation of the nerves in the neck and in the lumbosacral joints, and sagging ribs can stretch the nerves passing out from between the dorsal vertebrae!

In the sacral portion of the spine where there is no movement between the five segments of the sacrum, highly sensitive nerves are protected by openings of solid bone. But if all the nerves leaving the spinal column were so well-protected, we would be "stiff as a board."

In any event, if you keep your spine flexible, strong, and erect, there is little chance of normal vertebrae "pinching" the nerves. Drill 4 under "Four Beneficial Posture Drills" in Chapter 9, as well as many of the exercises in Chapter 12, will keep your spine loosened up.

Actually, very little movement takes place between any two vertebrae (about one-eighth of an inch to be exact), but the total amount of movement over the entire length of the spinal column adds up to considerable flexibility. When a vertebra moves too far, the spinal joints may be strained, or they may bind or lock in an abnormal position (subluxation). In either case, there is a great deal of pain, so you do not have to worry about your vertebrae being "out of place" without your knowing about it.

When general misalignment of the spinal column occurs because of poor posture, you will have to strengthen your muscles and improve your posture to eliminate the aches and pains caused by the vertebrae sagging against their ligaments; but when a single vertebra locks or binds to cause pain during an awkward movement, it can be treated effectively by manipulation.

But do not worry. With a dense array of ligaments and interlocking joints guarding the movement of your spinal column, your spinal cord is completely safe from injury unless you "break your back" in a severe accident of some sort.

The Muscles in Your Back

The ligaments and discs binding the vertebrae together do not have any power of contraction, so the spine must be held erect and put into motion by muscles. There are about 80 muscles covering the back, some of which reach from the top to the bottom of the vertebral column. Doctors usually refer to the muscles involved in holding the spine erect as "spina erecta muscles."

Nothing is more mysterious or fascinating than the function of layer after layer of back muscles that carry us around in an erect posture. Consider the act of walking, for example. When we shift our weight from one foot to the other in balancing the bodyweight for each step, there must be simultaneous contraction and relaxation of dozens of different muscles around the spine—and the contractions are so smooth and well-timed that we do not feel a thing or give it a second thought; that is, of course, if we do not have back trouble. When something does go wrong in the back or spine, the slightest movement can be agonizing. Ask any back sufferer.

Actually, just about all of the muscles of the trunk are involved in holding the spine erect. The muscles of the chest, for example, support the rib cage on the spine, while the abdominal muscles aid in supporting the spine in front. Even the muscles of the hips lend a hand in keeping the foundation of the spine level. This is why the exercises in Chapters 12 and 13 are so general.

Proper exercise for all of the muscles supporting the spine directly or indirectly would afford a high degree of protection for the spinal joints, and it would aid in preventing such common muscular disorders as lumbago or myositis (muscular inflammation).

There are a number of painful conditions occurring in and around back muscles that are not necessarily related to disorders of the spinal joints. But the muscles and joints are so closely related that muscle spasm can cause joint pain, and joint pain can cause muscle spasm.

Thus, by keeping the muscles of your back in good shape, you will be less likely to experience that vicious circle of muscle-joint pain that plagues so many poorly conditioned persons.

UNSEEN CAUSES OF BACK TROUBLE

Because of the extremely complex nature of the closely related structures of the back and spine, your doctor may not always know what is causing your back trouble. For example, trouble can develop in the cartilage covering the bone and joint surfaces, in the capsules (synovial sacs) covering and lubricating the joints, in the muscle fibers, in the sheets of tissue covering and separating the muscles, in the tendons, and in many other hidden structures of the back—not to mention the ligaments and discs. Trouble may also develop in bursae (lubricating sacs) that are sometimes found between large muscles that must move over bone or rub against each other.

Since routine X-ray examination does not reveal the soft tissues of any of these structures, it is no wonder that the cause of many a backache lies in the shadow of the unknown.

The Germans used to refer to acute back pain that comes on suddenly for no known reason as "hexenschusz," or a "witches' shot."

Fortunately, most back troubles not caused by infection, bone disease, tumors, or disc herniation are not serious, and they usually respond to physical treatment. Most of them, in fact, could be prevented with proper attention to exercise, correct lifting techniques, and improved working conditions. In many cases, an on-the-job backache that cannot be associated with any obvious violation of the rules of back care other than prolonged sitting or standing can be relieved simply by taking the rest-break exercises described in Chapter 10.

So even when a doctor does not know what is causing your backache, you can very often find relief in simple home-treatment and prevention techniques.

It's Not "All in Your Head"

Considering all the causes of backache that are hidden from view or detection, it is obvious that not every undiagnosed backache is a figment of the patient's imagination. There are, of course, many nervous and psychological causes of backache, but it is sometimes impossible to draw a definite line between backaches of physical origin and backaches of nervous origin.

Not too many years ago, before a great deal was learned about the spine, persons who had a backache that did not fit into any one of several major and somewhat serious categories were very often suspected of "putting on" or malingering, or of being a hypochondriac. This was especially true in the armed forces. And many a "dog-face" who complained of backache after carrying a heavy pack on a 10-mile hike was accused of "goofing off" because he did not have symptoms of some textbook malady.

No doubt, there were—and still are—many lazy people who feign back trouble to avoid unpleasant duties. But today we know that many formerly unrecognized causes of backache were probably overlooked as being "phony." And there are probably still many causes of backache that have not yet been uncovered. I have had many patients, for example, who were cured of chronic backache by manipulation of the vertebrae, even when the cause of the backache was not obvious.

But the point is that every backache has a cause, whether it is physical or emotional in origin. So you do not have to sit down and twiddle your thumbs just because your doctor cannot find a cause for your backache.

If you have an unrelieved chronic backache that is not being caused by any known or serious disturbance, then there is a possibility that it might be resulting from physical weakness or structural irritation that could be corrected by exercise and improved posture.

I knew a sedentary school teacher who had developed a postural slump that gave him a constant backache during the day. When he lay down at night his backache would be relieved for a while, but it would begin again each morning before the alarm went off. So he usually had to get out of bed around 4 a.m. to relieve his backache, which would begin again around 10 a.m. And this had been going on for several years! Since repeated medical examination had failed to find any obvious structural or organic disorder, he was usually told that his trouble was "just tension." I told him how to firm up his bed and then instructed him in postural exercises, as well as in the self-help measures described under "The Backache of All-Day Sitting or Standing" in Chapter 8. After several weeks, his backache was gone, and he told me one day with a broad smile, "Doc, for the first time in years, I'm enjoying my work. And for the first time in years, I sleep until my alarm clock goes off." I could not have been more pleased.

But remember that emotional tension is also a common cause

of backache. So make every effort to maintain a tranquil mind from day to day—and be sure to read Chapter 11 on "What to Do About Nervous Backache."

"BACK TROUBLE" THAT ISN'T BACK TROUBLE

As if an attempt by nature to make things more complicated in the diagnosis and treatment of back trouble, there are a number of internal (organic) disorders that refer their symptoms back over nerves, through connector fibers, to the spinal nerves where the pain is felt in the back.

Gall bladder disease, for example, can cause pain in the area of the right shoulder blade. Kidney trouble can cause a dull backache at the bottom of the rib cage in back. Bladder disorders can cause low backache, while hemorrhoids can cause sacral backache. Diseases of the lungs, the diaphragm, or the aorta (the large artery leaving the heart) can cause pain up around the base of the neck. Women with "female trouble" and men with prostate trouble almost always have low backache. And, of course, there are many organic diseases that can cause backache at the level of the disturbance.

A man once came into my office complaining of back pain, but he would not tell me where it was or what it felt like. "You find it, Doc," he said, "and tell me what my trouble is."

I would not ordinarily accept a patient who would "test" a doctor by withholding information, but because I detected a trace of fear and apprehension in the man's face I examined his spine from top to bottom with simple mechanical procedures. I could not find anything wrong with his spine, and when I told him this I could tell by the look on his face that he thought I had missed an obvious cause for his back pain.

"If you can't find it," he said, "you can't treat it."

He did tell me where the pain was, however, and he said that it was being caused by a certain vertebra that was out of line. When I finally convinced him that the pain he described and the condition of his spine did not add up to back trouble, and that the pain might be coming from a diseased organ, he admitted that a radiologist had told him just the day before that he had some kind of growth in his stomach that should be removed surgically. "But I didn't believe him," he said, "because my back was hurting worse than my stomach. So I figured that my back must be out of place. I've had trouble with it before, and my doctor told me that my stomach vertebra was slipping out of place."

I assured the frightened man that there are many organic diseases that can make a normal back hurt, and I suggested that he return to the hospital for further examination. When the tumor was removed, his back pain disappeared.

Many infectious conditions, such as influenza or tonsillitis, can cause severe backache. Diseases of the nervous system, such as disseminated sclerosis or Parkinson's disease, can cause backache in the early stages of their development—and the list could go on and on.

In any event, serious infectious diseases such as polio or meningitis cause many symptoms that are more obvious than backache, so you do not need to worry about being seriously ill every time you have a simple backache. When you do develop a backache that is accompanied by fever and other symptoms of illness, see your doctor.

Any kind of back pain that does not seem to disturb movement of the muscles or bones in the back should be suspected of having an internal origin until medical examination proves otherwise. As a general rule, you will feel pain in your back when you bend your spine, when you use your arms or legs, when you cough, when you get up and down from a chair, when you turn over in bed, or during other physical stresses if it is your back or spine that is at fault.

There are, of course, a few organic diseases that sometimes cause a reflex spasm of abdominal or back muscles that will pull the spine over to one side; and if this spasm is prolonged, it may cause joint symptoms that will make it difficult for your doctor to evaluate your trouble without running basic laboratory tests. In most cases, however, muscle spasm that is triggered by back trouble will release when you lie down, whereas the muscle spasm and pain triggered by organic disease will persist regardless of the posture you assume. Of course, if you should suffer a serious spinal injury, muscle spasm may persist in all postures for a few days, and simple movement of the spine in any direction will be painful. In this case, the cause of your trouble will be obvious. But if symptoms of any kind persist long after the injury occurred, you should return to your doctor for additional examination to eliminate the possibility that some other disturbance may have occurred as a result of or apart from the injury.

BACK TROUBLE IN DISGUISE

Just as an organ can "refer" pain into the structures of the back, the spinal column can refer pain into other parts of the body. As I mentioned earlier, there are spinal nerves (31 pairs) passing out from between the vertebrae on both sides of the vertebral column. When one of these nerves is irritated or pressed upon in its exit from the spine (where it branches out from the spinal cord), the symptoms of the irritation may be referred into the structure supplied by the nerve. If a nerve is irritated in the lower portion of the spine, for example, there may be pain, numbness, and other symptoms in the portion of the thigh or leg corresponding to the segment of the spine where the irritation is taking place.

When a nerve is irritated in the middle of your spine, you may feel the pain somewhere around the front of your chest. And if a nerve is pinched or irritated in your neck, the pain will radiate into your head, shoulder, or arm. This does not mean, however, that there is anything wrong with the structures where you feel the pain. All of your trouble may be in the disturbed spinal joints, *even though you may not feel a thing in your back.* It is not at all uncommon for persons with nerve pain in a leg to apply treatment to the leg itself. I talked to one man, for example, who used salves, plasters, liniments, epsom salts, bandages, laxatives, and other remedies before he found out his leg pain was coming from his back.

Like a telephone line that contains wires leading to and from the receiver, a spinal nerve contains fibers coming from and going to the body structure it supplies. Thus, if irritation takes place on the back side of the nerve, there may be pain, numbness, loss of sensation, and other sensory disturbances in the skin over the area supplied by the nerve. If the irritation takes place on the front side of the nerve, however, there may be muscle weakness or localized paralysis (as in polio). This is why two people may have different symptoms, even though the same nerve and joint are involved.

In any event, when the spinal nerves are "pinched," there does not seem to be much danger of organic disease occurring as a result. Spinal nerves, for example, supply such body structures as muscles and skin, while the internal organs are supplied by a separate nervous system (sympathetic and parasympathetic) whose centers are located outside the spinal column. There are, of course, fibers connecting these two systems, which accounts for the fact that pain originating in the structures of the back and spine can sometimes be referred into the vicinity of an organ. Very bad body mechanics can sometimes irritate important nerve centers in the neck and in the thoracic and abdominal cavities to cause disturbances in the functions of the various organs.

Many years ago, before the nature of "referred pain" was fully understood, many unnecessary operations were performed by surgeons who thought that an undiagnosed abdominal pain might be a hidden organic disease; and many bonesetters who relieved such pain by manipulating the joints thought that they had cured an organic disease.

Summary

1. Your spine and its supporting muscles are very complicated structures; but if you have a basic knowledge of how they work, you will be able to make better use of procedures recommended for correction and prevention of back trouble. Furthermore, by being familiar with the structures of your spine, you can eliminate unnecessary worry about some of the "bumps" you feel in your back, and you will have a better idea of what is or is not normal in the appearance of your back.

2. Since many organic diseases refer pain into the structures of the back, get a good medical checkup when you have back pain that seems to be unaffected by bending and twisting of your spine. And when you have a pain somewhere in your body for which no organic cause can be found, have your spine examined. Your trouble could be referred pain from a spinal joint, which could possibly be corrected by manipulation.

3. Do not worry about your vertebrae getting "out of place" and pinching your spinal nerves without you knowing about it. This will not happen unless you suffer an injury

or unless your spine is diseased; and if it does happen, you will experience pain, numbness, or some other obvious and disturbing symptom.

4. Since the pull of gravity tends to exaggerate the normal curves of the spine, try to lie down occasionally during the day in order to relieve the pressure on your joints and discs.

5. If you do not have any serious back trouble at the present time, you might not absorb much of the material describing the spine. But when back pain strikes, as it may do at any time like a bolt of lightning, you will want to know all about the structures affected. For this reason, you will probably want to read portions of this chapter again at a later date.

4

Some Major Causes of
Low-Back Trouble

If you have read the first three chapters closely, you already know a great deal about what causes backache in general; and if you have retained any of the information describing the structures of the back and spine, you should be able to visualize many of the things that might go wrong to cause a backache.

You do not have to be a trained professional to be knowledgeable about your own back and spine. You can be just as well informed about back care as a teenager can be about hot rods. So do not throw up your hands in despair just because there is not one cause and one cure for every type of backache. When your doctor tells you that you have a slipped disc, a lumbosacral strain, a sacroiliac strain, coccygodynia, fibrositis, or a muscle spasm, you will have some idea of what he is talking about after you have read this chapter. And if you make use of the recommended measures of treatment and prevention as outlined throughout this book, you will find self-help simple enough and effective.

Fortunately, most back trouble is simply the result of strain or fatigue, which is often secondary to bad working postures and poor muscle tone. But as you will learn in a moment, there are a number of bony abnormalities that are commonly present in the spine from birth, and these may make it easier to strain or injure the back. Of course, even when the spinal joints are not normal, there is less chance of strain if posture is good and if correct lifting techniques are observed.

How to Recognize the Symptoms of Strain

Simple strain can, of course, occur anywhere in the back, but it is most common in the lower back.

When a strain is minor, it may not cause much trouble until 12 to 24 hours after the actual strain, since it may take that long for enough swelling to build up around the injured tissues or joints to cause stiffness, pressure, and pain. As a result, many people fail to associate a slight injury one day with acute back-ache the following day.

An office worker, for example, who felt a little pain in his back when he pushed his desk across the room, felt "all right" for the rest of the day. But when he got up the next morning, his back was so sore and stiff that he could hardly get around. He could not understand why his back was hurting!

A secretary who was working late in a badly lighted room in an effort to finish up a lengthy typing assignment had to lean to her left to read her copy material. After a couple of hours, she complained of a little backache. "It's nothing," she said. She went home, prepared supper, and went to bed with only a small amount of discomfort. The next morning, however, she was not able to return to work. She did not know what had caused her backache.

These are typical examples of the *delayed reactions* of minor back strains that could have been prevented with a little informed caution. So be sure to observe all the back-care precautions you read about in this book, *no matter how simple they may seem to be.*

When a strain is more severe, there is usually a great deal of pain and disability at the time of the injury or immediately following the injury. A yard worker, for example, who was lifting a rented power mower into the trunk of his car, felt a sharp pain in his back. His disability was so acute that he could not stand up without help. He had strained the ligaments in his lower back.

A motorist who was trying to unhook two cars that had "locked bumpers" felt a sharp pain and a snap on one side of his back, and had to be carried home like a cripple. He had torn a back muscle.

A visiting relative had to call off a fishing trip after he inadvertently stepped off an unfamiliar split-level floor and injured the joints of his lumbar spine.

All of these injuries presented symptoms of acute strain, and, like most back strains, *they could have been prevented.*

In any event, back injuries that are serious enough to cause a great deal of immediate pain and disability can usually be counted on to result in at least one sleepless night. So if they do not respond to aspirin and cold or hot packs (see Chapter 7), you may need medication to get you through the first few days until the acuteness of the injury subsides; that is, if you want to sleep as usual. A throbbing backache that feels as if an army is marching over your back can give you a miserable night.

The lumbar and low-back portions of the spine are the most common sites of backache and back pain. For this reason, most of this chapter will be devoted to disorders of the lumbar, sacral, and coccygeal portions of the spine—how and why they occur. If you have back trouble, you might recognize your trouble in one of the descriptions to follow. You will also find many useful suggestions for treating and preventing specific low-back ailments.

The Most Common Back Injury: Lumbosacral Strain

The lumbosacral joints, which serve as "bottom man" for the entire spine, are the joints most often involved in low-back disorders, especially in adults. In addition to being a supporting pivot for the vertebral column, the lumbosacral joints are frequently the site of mechanical deformities. This is why they are so easily strained when abnormal stresses of any kind are placed on the spine. Poor posture, heavy or improper lifting, incorrect sleeping or sitting positions, excessive fatigue, and so on, are common causes of lumbosacral strain.

When the lumbosacral joints are acutely strained, it may be difficult or impossible to stand erect without the aid of a spine-splinting lumbosacral corset.

Whatever you might do to cause a lumbosacral strain, try to make sure that the strain is not repeated! Recurring strain of this type can result in a relaxation of the ligaments binding these joints together, thus resulting in "lumbosacral instability," which adds up to chronic back trouble.

In any kind of low-back trouble, there is a tendency for the knees to buckle when the spine is tilted in an awkward or un-balanced manner. This does not mean that you are in danger of being paralyzed. It is just nature's way of trying to relieve the stress on the affected joints.

Manipulation is sometimes helpful in "loosening up" lumbo-sacral joints that are locked in abnormal positions. Many people who have chronic lumbosacral trouble discover that they can "unlock" their back by hanging from a tree limb or by supporting their bodyweight on a pair of crutches. (See "Traction with a Chair" in Chapter 7.)

Although strong back muscles are important in preventing lumbosacral strain, most injuries of this type that I have seen have occurred as a result of improper lifting techniques.

THOSE PAINFUL SACROILIAC STRAINS

The sacroiliac joints, as you recall, are formed by the joining of the pelvis (iliac bones) to the sacrum on each side, and they are just below the lumbosacral joints.

Persons who suffer a locked sacroiliac joint for the first time usually "drop like a shot," and the pain is so severe that an am-bulance may be needed to cart the paralyzed patient off to a hospital. I know one man who locked a sacroiliac joint while in bed, and when it happened, he had one leg on the bed and one leg off the bed. And he stayed that way until a doctor arrived to give him a pain-killing injection! If this ever happens to you, re-gardless of where you are, call your family physician for medication. In many cases, the joint will unlock if you can be relieved of pain enough to move around a little.

Unlike lumbosacral strain in which the pain is usually felt in the center of the lower back, a sacroiliac strain is felt on one side of the back; that is, in the pelvic area near the hip. You can locate the sacroiliac joints by locating the dimples above the buttocks on each side.

Like lumbosacral strain, sacroiliac strain can occur in any kind of heavy or awkward lifting, but it occurs most often in movements that place off-center leverage, torsion, or twisting on the lower back. A secretary, for example, who sits on one buttock and then turns suddenly and vigorously to that side might strain the anchored sacroiliac joint on the same side. A worker who twists his body around to pick up a box and then turns with his bodyweight supported on one leg might suffer a sacroiliac strain. Anyone unaccustomed to toe-touching exercises could strain *both* sacroiliac joints by using forceful momentum in an effort to reach the toes while the knees are locked out straight. I have seen more than one "weekend athlete" who strained a sacroiliac joint by kicking a football or by swinging a golf club in "correct form."

If you do strain one of your sacroiliac joints, you might notice a little pain or aching in your groin. Men frequently complain of their testicles aching. This does not mean that they have ruptured themselves, however. What they are feeling is just "referred" pain (from the sacroiliac joints) of the type discussed in Chapter 3.

It is not possible, of course, to describe all the various ways that a sacroiliac joint can be strained. If you will just observe all the rules on exercise, posture, and correct lifting techniques outlined in other chapters of this book, you can greatly reduce your chances of suffering a sacroiliac strain.

Always bring persistent sacroiliac pain to the attention of your doctor. It is not unheard of for these joints to become infected with tuberculosis or rheumatoid arthritis.

What to Do About a "Slipped Disc"

A ruptured or "slipped" disc is a protrusion of the soft center of a disc from between two vertebrae, and it is one of the most serious mechanical disturbances commonly occurring in the spine, since it is an injury that may never completely heal. However, orthopedic specialists tell us that a large proportion of "slipped discs" will recover satisfactorily without surgery if prolonged conservative therapy is employed; that is, if manipulation, rest, heat, support, massage, traction, a firm bed, special exercises, and other physical treatments are used over a period of time. One well-known orthopedic surgeon estimated that 75 to 80 percent of patients treated conservatively for herniated intervertebral disc will respond to such treatment.

Thus, not every slipped disc will result in serious or permanent disability. In fact, one authority stated that just about everyone after the age of 40 will sustain at least one lumbar disc protrusion, but that not every disc protrusion will cause symptoms.

We are, of course, concerned only with those disc injuries that cause symptoms, and we want to avoid disc surgery whenever possible.

When slipped-disc symptoms do occur, the disc between the 5th lumbar vertebra and the sacrum (the last disc in the spine, at the lumbosacral joints) is the one most often involved, since it carries the greatest amount of weight. In a 200-pound man, for example, the bottom disc must support about 120 pounds, not to mention the additional weight of heavy objects that are lifted. This is one reason why your doctor always tells you to get rid of that "bay window" when you complain of low-back pain.

Your doctor can usually tell when surgery is needed for a slipped disc by observing the amount of nerve damage that takes place. When symptoms are severe and progressive, and unrelieved by conservative (home treatment) measures, neither the patient nor the doctor will have any trouble deciding about the need for surgery.

Fortunately, the greatest majority of diagnosed disc injuries seem to recover under physical treatment, as mentioned earlier; so no one who is not experiencing continuous pain or disability, or showing evidence of serious damage to nerve trunks, should hastily submit to surgery for removal of a suspected slipped disc, especially if relief can be obtained by rest and other measures.

Many suspected disc injuries are not disc injuries at all and will recover with time. In fact, a professor of surgery at Hamburg University in West Germany has recommended the use of manipulation for "disc injuries" that do not show *positive* evidence of complete herniation, since, as he put it, many cases diagnosed as herniated disc are, as surgery often reveals, not that at all. For this reason, surgery should always be a measure of last resort.

Disc herniation can, of course, occur anywhere in the spine. When it occurs above the level of the third lumbar vertebra (above the beltline) where the spinal cord ends (the spinal canal below this point is filled with a large number of nerve trunks that hang down from the end of the spinal cord like the hair on a horse's tail), there would be greater danger of spinal cord compression.

Fortunately, the intervertebral discs are normally very tough, and it takes a great deal of force or a severe injury to rupture a healthy disc. But when a disc is weak or defective, it may be ruptured rather easily when placed under awkward or heavy stresses. Sneezing, for example, when done while the body is bent forward, can rupture a weak disc. Always try to avoid lifting or straining while your spine is slumped if you want to prevent unnecessary compression of your discs.

Good posture, strong muscles, and proper lifting techniques are all important in protecting potentially weak discs.

Sciatica—The Pain That Puts Your Leg in a Vise

Sciatica is a leg pain radiating down the sciatic nerve; and since this nerve is made up of spinal nerves that branch out from between the lower lumbar vertebrae and the segments of the sacrum (to come together and form one large nerve that travels down the leg), pain radiating down the back of the thigh into the leg is usually caused by mechanical irritation of a nerve trunk somewhere in the lower spine.

The pain of sciatica can be sharp and severe, and it can make your leg feel as if its bones are being squeezed in a great vise. Although disc herniation is the most common cause of sciatica, it can also be caused by arthritis, lumbosacral strain, sacroiliac strain, bad posture, tumors, and other low-back disturbances. When sciatic pain accompanies joint strain, it will usually disappear along with the back symptoms after a few days. But when sciatic pain occurs with a disc injury, it may come and go long after acute back symptoms have subsided.

In any severe and progressive sciatic nerve pain for which no obvious cause can be found, your doctor might want to run special tests to eliminate the possibility of a tumor growing in the spinal canal. For the most part, however, the nerve pain of a disc injury will usually be relieved with rest or traction, whereas the pain caused by a tumor in the spinal canal may seem to get worse with rest.

Do not try to "wear out" a leg pain that is made worse by standing or sitting. If you keep pressure on the nerve by keeping weight on the disc, the nerve may swell up until it is larger than the opening it passes through. And when this happens, you will experience a constant leg pain that may require many weeks of rest and medication for recovery. Adequate rest at the very beginning, however, will prevent excessive irritation until the swelling in the injured tissues can subside; then, when you get back on your feet again, there may be adequate room for the nerve between the vertebrae, and your period of disability may be shortened considerably. *So always rest when you have a leg pain that is made worse by sitting or standing.*

Persons who have repeated recurrences of sciatic nerve pain that is being caused by a slipped disc or by an arthritic condition can usually benefit by using spinal traction at home. Although most people have hospital insurance that will cover a stay in the hospital, it is usually more convenient to use traction at home whenever possible. (See "How to Rig Up Traction at Home" in Chapter 7.)

An automobile mechanic, for example, who was under the shadow of a surgeon's scalpel for ruptured disc, reports that every time his right leg begins to feel "numb and tingly" he rigs up his traction and stretches his spine for an hour or so a couple of times a day. It has been five years since his fifth lumbar disc ruptured, and he maintains that the traction is still effective in preventing a recurrence of his leg pain. Not everyone will be so lucky, but such home treatment is certainly worth a try if your doctor will go along with it.

Since most sciatic nerve pains occur from irritation of the nerve at the opening on the back of the spine where it passes out to the leg, try lying on your side and rounding your lower back by gently pulling your knees up toward your chest to relieve your symptoms.

Once recovery from a "pinched" sciatic nerve has taken place, good posture that is maintained by well-toned back muscles will be important in keeping the vertebrae in proper alignment for free passage of the nerves.

LORDOSIS—THE SWAY-BACKED BACKACHE

Lordosis, or "sway back," is an exaggeration of the normal lumbar curve—that is, the curve of the lower back is greatly increased. Although there are many cases in which the lumbar spine is sway-backed because of structural characteristics in the spine, most sway-backs develop because of bad posture.

In the normal spine in which the spinal curves are balanced, the bodyweight is supported primarily on the discs, but when a sway-backed condition develops, the joints of the lumbar spine began to assume the function of weight bearing and a shearing strain is placed on the lumbosacral joints. Furthermore, there may be a tendency for the bony spinous processes projecting back from the vertebrae to move closer together (as in closing the fingers of your hand), thus causing trouble as they rub together ("kissing spine").

A sway-backed spine by itself can cause backache, and if it is accompanied by other low-back disorders (such as joint defects), your troubles may be compounded.

One of the most persistent backaches I ever saw occurred in an overweight female who was a short-order cook in a busy cafe. She was extremely sway-backed, and her abdomen was so heavy and pendulous that she had to lean backward slightly in order to balance her bodyweight. She had a "pregnant woman's backache" that was greatly aggravated by her sway-backed spine. Postural exercises helped, but she did not get rid of her backache until she lost a great deal of weight.

If you do have a sway back, you should attempt correction with improved posture and exercise (Chapters 9 and 12). In the meantime, relief from the fatigue and stress of a sway back can be obtained by lying down on your side and pulling your knees up toward your chest, or by bowing your back backward to reverse the forward curve. Concentrate on standing tall in order to keep your spine from sagging, and tuck your hips under a little in order to flatten out your lower back.

Try to avoid activities in which you must lean backward. Painting a ceiling, hanging out a big wash on a high clothesline, or walking in a pair of high-heeled shoes, for example, can aggravate symptoms caused by a sway-backed spine. And sleeping face-down can cause acute backache.

As in any postural abnormality, strong supporting muscles are important in the care and prevention of sway back—and good posture is imperative.

SPONDYLOLISTHESIS—THE WANDERING VERTEBRA

When this condition occurs, the 5th lumbar vertebra (the last vertebra in the lumbar spine) slips forward over the sacrum (the bone fitted between the two pelvic bones), supporting and carrying the spine with it.

You have probably never even heard of spondylolisthesis, but, while it is not the most common cause of backache, anatomists say that the defect is present in 1 to 4 percent of all the skeletons they have studied.

When a vertebra does slip far enough to be classified as "Grade 2" or more, a patient's description of the disorder may lead the doctor to suspect the presence of a spondylolisthesis before X-ray examination reveals the abnormality. A 23-year-old female, for example, described her symptoms this way: "Doctor, my back feels like it is caving in, and both of my legs ache. My husband says that since I've gained weight, I've gotten a little shorter. Is this possible? And he says there is a little hollow in my lower back that wasn't there when he married me."

X-ray examination revealed a pronounced spondylolisthesis. Fortunately, this disorder does not always cause serious trouble, since the disc and the ligaments are usually strong enough to keep the vertebra from slipping too far.

Postural exercises, physical therapy, and a lumbosacral corset may relieve symptoms when the disorder is mild, but if there is a progressive increase in pain (especially leg pain), or if acute back pain recurs from time to time, an operation may be performed in which the "loose" vertebra is securely fixed to the vertebra below, thus locking it in position and permanently relieving the symptoms.

Excessive exercise or heavy lifting may aggravate the condition, so those who have such defects should try to work and exercise without putting too much weight on the lower back. *Falls or jumping from a height should be especially guarded against.*

Transitional Lumbosacral Joints—The Confused Vertebra

A transitional lumbosacral joint is quite the reverse of spondylolisthesis, in that the joint surface is excessive rather than deficient. An incompletely developed fifth lumbar vertebra, for example, is partially attached to the sacrum (either by growth of bone to bone or by extra joints) in such a way that it appears that the two bones attempted to grow together but failed. This abnormal attachment can occur on one or both sides. When it occurs on only one side, the opposite side is subjected to excessive strain brought about by one-sided movement of the defective vertebra. Also, the extra joints (which are actually abnormal bony growths fitted against each other) that may be found in this condition are almost always on a horizontal plane. Thus, they are forced to bear the brunt of excessive or abnormal weight bearing. With each step, for example, these joints may bang together like two blocks, resulting in a difficult-to-treat arthritis.

When abnormal development does take place in the lumbosacral joints, it may or may not cause trouble, and even then not usually until late in life. Occasionally, however, such defects will result in a puzzling form of backache in young people. A 19-year-old mill worker, for example, was fired from his job because constant complaining about his backache led his foreman to suspect him of "gold-bricking." When the young fellow came in for examination, he described his backache as a vague form of "soreness and weakness" that plagued him constantly, although he could move about normally. X-ray examination revealed a transitional fifth lumbar vertebra.

The lumbosacral portion of the spine must support about ten times more weight than the knee joint, so it will be important to observe correct lifting procedures and to maintain good posture, especially if you are having low-back trouble or if you know that you have bone defects in your lower spine.

SPINA BIFIDA—CLEFT SPINE

In the fetal development of your vertebral column, a projection of bone normally grows back from the vertebra on each side and then comes together in the back to form a bony ring for passage and protection of the spinal cord. When this growth or fusion is complete, the spinous process, a finger-like projection of bone on the back of each vertebra, is formed. As you learned in Chapter 3, these processes are evident visually in thin persons as bony bumps up and down the center of the back.

When spina bifida occurs, incomplete growth or fusion of one or more of these processes results in an open split or cleft on the back of the spine, leaving the spinal canal open except for the protection of overlying muscles and soft tissues. For some unknown reason, this defect, as a cause of backache, occurs more frequently in the lumbosacral portion of the spine where structural integrity is most important.

Persons suffering from backache caused by spina bifida complications should avoid backward bending and other activities that seem to cause back pain. It may be necessary to avoid pressing the lower back against hard surfaces, as in lying on a floor or leaning back against a fence rail.

In severe cases in which simple treatment does not relieve the symptoms, surgery may be performed to remove the sharp, bony projections—or the involved vertebrae may be fused together.

COCCYGODYNIA—THE PAINFUL TAILBONE

As you already know, the coccyx or "tail bone" seems to serve no useful purpose other than an attachment site for a few small muscles. The bone itself, however, is jointed to the sacrum by ligaments and has small bursae (lubricating sacs) surrounding its movable segments. Thus, it is possible to have "tailbone bursitis" that is similar to the bursitis we have in our shoulder.

This pain, however, is probably caused by strain resulting from the injuries and pressures suffered in falls and improper sitting. A business man, for example, who "sat on his spine" on a steel folding chair during a three-day business convention developed a tailbone pain that was so severe that he had to have his family physician give him injections in the painful area so that he could "keep going." It took him several months to get over his pain and disability, and during this time he had great difficulty in walking, sitting, and getting in and out of a chair. So try to sit erect and keep the pressure off that tailbone whenever possible. Most tailbone sufferers I know exemplify pure misery.

Patients with a painful tailbone are usually advised to sit on a doughnut-shaped rubber cushion so that no outside pressure will be placed against the bottom of the spine. Do not be embarrassed about carrying one of these ring-like cushions around to sit on. I know a hypochondriac who carries her cushion around as though it were the ultimate in status symbols.

Chairs and other sitting surfaces should be firm so that the bodyweight will not sink into the cushion and cause painful spreading of the buttocks, which can result in direct pressure against the coccyx. Special belts are sometimes used to strap the buttocks together to assure adequate protection for the coccyx when sitting.

Hot baths, hot packs, and other forms of heat, followed by light massage over the tailbone, might help. When pain is acute, however, cold packs might provide more immediate relief (see Chapter 7). Occasionally, manipulation through the rectum will be necessary, especially if there has been any forward displacement of the coccyx from falls or blows.

In most cases, time and conservative care will relieve the symptoms of painful tailbone, but there are occasions when injections or surgical removal of the coccyx may be necessary.

Pilonidal Sinus—The Draining Hair Pocket

The pilonidal sinus is an extremely disagreeable—though not serious—disorder. Occurring most often near the tailbone, the sinus is believed to be a folding in of the skin from improper development in the fetus, and it drains a foul-smelling secretion that is formed by infection and irritation in the airless pocket beneath the skin.

Although the sinus is present from birth, it does not usually begin to cause trouble until body secretions and hair growth are accelerated by the sexual changes of puberty. The pocket and its sinus (opening), which usually contains a growth of hair, can be removed surgically with little or no trouble; so it would be foolish for anyone to put up with the discomfort and bother of this disorder. I know a very lovely woman who kept her sinus "secret" because she was too embarrassed to submit to surgical care.

Boys and girls who may be too timid to reveal the presence of a pilonidal sinus should be inspected after puberty and then be encouraged to bring such a disorder to the attention of the family physician.

WHAT TO DO ABOUT MUSCLE SPASM

Muscle spasm can, of course, occur anywhere in the back. But since it most often occurs as a reaction to disturbances in the spine, it is most common in the lumbar portion of the back where spinal trouble is most common. In almost every case of acute back trouble involving the lower spine, for example, there will be a certain amount of muscle spasm that is designed by nature to "splint" the spine and protect it from further injury. The spasm is usually intensified when standing up, and relieved when lying down.

Although nature means well in providing reflex muscle spasm in joint and muscle injuries, prolonged or aggravated muscle spasm can make things worse by interfering with blood circulation and by jamming the injured joints together, thus increasing the severity of the spasm. Also, a muscle in continuous spasm releases waste products that are not removed by the hindered blood circulation.

Thus, *if rest, moist heat, and massage are not employed to stimulate the circulation of blood and to aid in the removal of waste products and accumulating tissue fluids, the muscle becomes inflamed and irritated and the spasm becomes worse.* This is one reason why you should rest when muscle spasm is triggered by standing and sitting erect.

A post-office employee who sorted mail several hours a day in unrelieved sitting and standing postures, for example, developed "lumbago" in the muscles of his lower back. Although the muscle soreness was mild at first, it grew progressively worse as the days passed. And since the Christmas mail rush had started, he did not want to ask for a few days off; in fact, he even worked a little overtime for the extra pay. He slept on a heating pad at night, and he took aspirin, but this did not seem to help. After five or six days, the affected muscles became painful and spastic, so he took a few pain-killer pills in order to keep working. After two weeks had passed, he could not even get relief by staying in bed. *It never occurred to him to try moist heat and massage,* however, and when I explained to him the techniques of using these simple self-help measures (see Chapter 7), he tried them and experienced some immediate relief. After three days, he was back at work.

If you suffer from a similar disorder, you can avoid letting your back get into such bad shape by taking a day or two off from work and using the same techniques of applying moist heat and massage.

One of the most fearsome-looking muscle spasms resulting from a spinal injury is the so-called "sciatic scoliosis," a temporary "S"-shaped spinal curvature brought about by the spasm of muscles on one side of the spine. If a nerve is being pinched on one side of the vertebral column, for example, reflex muscle spasm may pull the spine to the opposite side in order to widen the opening through which the nerve is passing. In certain types of joint injuries, however, the spasm may pull the spine toward the injured side in order to prevent movement in the joint and to relieve painful traction on the injured tissues.

Treatment, of course, should be directed toward the injury as well as toward the spasm. Rest and other home-treatment techniques will usually do the job. But if muscle spasm should persist in spite of everything you do, your family physician can prescribe muscle-relaxing and pain-killing drugs that will allow the muscle to relax, thus giving it an opportunity to restore its normal circulation and to break the vicious cycle of pain and spasm.

Muscle spasms resulting from injury to the muscles or the spine can, of course, be prevented by keeping your back strong and then using it correctly.

THE MUSCLE INFLAMMATION OF FIBROMYOSITIS

Fibromyositis, sometimes called "fibrositis" or "myositis," is a muscle inflammation that can cause muscle spasm and a variety of other symptoms that may resemble just about any kind of back trouble. There are many causes of this type of muscle pain, but the three most common causes can be eliminated with a little intelligent caution.

Everyone will occasionally experience a backache that is caused by muscular inflammation, so the preventive techniques outlined below should be an important part of your back-care program.

Eliminating Causes of Fibromyositis

(1) *Fatigue and weak muscles* are probably the most common causes of fibromyositis. When a muscle is weak, of course, it fatigues more rapidly; but even strong muscles become fatigued when placed under the continuous tension of prolonged awkward and static postures that do not allow full and free movement. An assembly-line worker, for example, who must hover over the same limited task day after day may finish each day with a back-breaking backache that lingers to some extent even over the weekends. (See "Overcoming Backache at the End of the Day" in Chapter 8.)

What happens, of course, is that the continuous tension on the muscles in the unchanging posture interferes with the circulation of blood to such an extent that the waste products generated by the muscle tension accumulate to cause muscle inflammation.

The obvious solution to the aches and pains of static postures would be to take frequent breaks during the day (if a job change is not possible) so that the muscles can be put through a full and varied range of movement in order to pump blood through the muscles, thus flushing out the waste products of fatigue.

Muscle tension caused by prolonged nervous tension can also cause fibromyositis, so try to get away from the tension of the home or office for a few hours each day. I have seen housewives, business executives, TV personalities, and college presidents alike come down periodically with myositis or muscle inflammation (usually around the neck and shoulders) when heavy and continuous work loads resulted in constant and unbearable tension.

Heat and massage may relieve the symptoms of muscle inflammation, but its cure and prevention lie in movement and exercise as well as in good posture and on-the-job relaxation. (See "Relaxing on the Job" in Chapter 11.)

If you have a job in which you are not able to move around very much, you should occasionally exercise your muscles and loosen up your joints right on the job by putting all of your joints through a full range of movement. (See "Five Simple Rest-Break Exercises" in Chapter 10.)

(2) *Exposure to cold* is another common cause of muscle inflammation, and it happens most often in individuals who sleep and work under the direct air currents of fans, ventilators, and air conditioners.

A clerk, for example, who got extremely hot cleaning out a cluttered store room, sat down to rest with a large fan blowing against his bare back. A few hours later, his entire back began to get a little stiff, and by morning his neck and lower back were painfully locked with muscle spasm. I have seen a number of patients who developed myositis after lying on cold ground or floors.

The application of hot packs, followed by massage, will usually relieve the symptoms of this type of myositis, but it should be prevented by avoiding muscle chills, especially when the muscles are overheated from hot weather or exercise. If you perspire heavily during work or exercise, wear enough clothing to keep your muscles from being cooled suddenly, and then wait until you "cool off" before you go into a cold, air conditioned room.

(3) *Excessive heat* that causes a great deal of sweating is another common cause of back pain among laborers, especially if the salt and water lost by profuse sweating are not replaced by drinking water and taking salt tablets right on the job. When you lose too much salt by sweating, the chemical balance in the muscles is disturbed, so that when they become fatigued they cramp, go into spasm, or just ache. So if you have a job that calls for heavy labor and a great deal of sweating, make sure that there is plenty of drinking water and salt tablets handy.

A football player who tried to "toughen up" by practicing long hours in full uniform without drinking water suffered severe cramps with nausea after scrimmaging. All he had to do to prevent a recurrence of the cramps was to drink a little water when he felt he needed it.

Thirst should never be denied, for any reason, when water is available—and this goes as much for fat people who exercise for weight reduction as for well-conditioned athletes.

Persons who perspire heavily in work or athletics can prevent the muscle spasm of dehydration by drinking a .1 percent salt solution or by taking one salt tablet with every 6 ounces of water during work periods.

OTHER CAUSES OF BACK TROUBLE

There are, of course, many other causes of low-back trouble, some of which will be discussed in other chapters in this book. Arthritis and spinal curvatures, for example, are fairly common causes of backache, but since these are conditions affecting the entire spine, they are covered in Chapter 6.

BONE DISEASE—DON'T TAKE YOUR BACK PAIN FOR GRANTED

It is always easier for your doctor to diagnose the cause of your back pain when it occurs as the result of a strain or injury. But rarely an accident that appears to injure the back will stir up symptoms in an early and undetected bone disease. One man, for example, who "strained" his back lifting a boat motor, felt sure that his increasingly severe back pain was the result of the strain. X-ray examination revealed bone cancer.

Thus, any persistent back pain should not be shrugged off as being a "strain" just because it started with an injury.

If you may have a history of tuberculosis, venereal disease, or cancer, be sure to tell your doctor about it when you are being examined for persistent back pain. Any of these diseases can infect the spine. Cancer, for example, sometimes spreads from the breast, the prostate gland, the thyroid gland, the kidneys, or the lungs to the vertebrae. Sarcoma, another bone disease resembling carcinoma, can originate in the spine; but cancer, which is more common, usually spreads to the spine from some other part of the body.

Summary

1. Simple strains of the spine and its supporting structures

are the most common cause of acute back pain, but chronic backache is very often complicated by bony defects that have existed in the spine from birth.

2. Because of the frequent involvement of the sciatic nerve in the lower lumbar spine where most of our back trouble develops, it is important to take every possible precaution in guarding against low-back injury. The preventive measures in Part II of this book will be of special importance in taking care of your lower back.

3. If you already have back trouble that fits any of the disorders discussed in this chapter, make use of the suggestions accompanying the description of your disorder (according to the instructions in Chapter 7 when possible), and then make prevention a part of your treatment.

4. Even if you do not now suffer from any of the disorders described in this chapter, be sure to read the complete chapter anyway so that you will learn how to *prevent* these disorders when possible!

5. You can "slip a disc," strain a sacroiliac joint, sprain your lumbosacral joints, or "pull a muscle" by violating any of the rules of correct lifting techniques (Chapter 10).

6. Do not sneeze while you are bent over or supporting a weight, lest you rupture a weak disc.

7. If you are sway-backed, avoid activities in which you must bend backward. Occasionally lie down on your side and round-out your lower back by pulling your knees up toward your chest.

8. Do not permit chilling of a muscle by direct exposure to the cooling drafts of a fan or an air conditioner, especially when you are perspiring. If you do suffer a muscle spasm from such exposure, simple moist heat and massage are usually the best treatment.

9. Avoid excessive fatigue in work or activities that you are not accustomed to, especially if your muscles are weak from lack of exercise.

10. Always drink a lot of water and take salt tablets when you are working long hours on a job that causes you to sweat profusely.

5

Common Causes of Back
Trouble Above
the Waistline

Many of the disorders causing low-back trouble—such as "slipped disc"—can, of course, occur in other portions of the spine. But, as in the lower back, simple strain and fatigue resulting from overexertion and postural strain are probably the most common causes of back trouble above the waistline. There are, however, several disorders occurring primarily in the upper portions of the back and spine that warrant special attention.

In addition to explaining the causes of many common disorders that can occur in your upper back, this chapter also contains many simple suggestions for preventing the development of backache, as well as many self-help suggestions in the care of specific disorders.

THE TRIANGLE BACKACHE (SCAPULOCOSTAL SYNDROME)

Deep, sickening pain very often occurs in the muscles in the

66

triangular area between the shoulder blade, the spine, and the base of the neck (on one side of the back) from simple postural strains in persons who have round shoulders and a drooping shoulder girdle. When the posture is bad and the muscles are weak, many vague aches and pains occur in the muscles that must hold the body erect against the relentless pull of gravity. And muscle spasms frequently occur in muscles that are subjected to one-sided postural strains.

Most of these symptoms respond to heat, massage, and postural exercises, but you should also try to *avoid using large pillows or a large number of small pillows under your head when you are sleeping on your back.* A bed that is too soft and a pillow that is too thick will nullify the effects of the postural exercises you take during the day.

There are some people who develop the very bad habit of propping their head up with such thick pillows (sometimes to watch TV) that their neck is curved sharply upwards during sleep. If this is one of your faults, gradually lower your pillow until your head and neck are in line with the rest of your spine.

I have seen a number of patients who complain of neck and "shoulder" trouble (in the triangular area where the neck joins the shoulder) but who say that they cannot sleep without using two pillows. In other words, they find it difficult to change a bad habit, even when it is a cause of physical distress. It has also been my observation that a number of people who suffer from chronic stiffness at the bottom of the neck use foam-rubber pillows. For this reason, I have wondered if the springy nature of such pillows keeps the neck muscles tense from lack of firm support. If you have a chronic stiff neck and you use a rubber pillow, try changing to a solidly packed feather pillow and see if it will help.

Pain Between the Shoulder Blades
(Interscapular Backache)

Most of the causes of muscle pain, as well as many spinal disorders, can cause pain between the shoulder blades; but exposure to cold and dampness, poor posture, weak muscles, fatigue, strain, and muscle inflammation would probably head the list. Fortunately, all of these respond to physical treatment, and all of them can be prevented.

Postural exercises—that is, exercises designed to strengthen the muscles responsible for holding the body erect—are probably the most important part of prevention and cure for muscle pain in the upper back.

I knew a barber, for example, who suffered from such severe pain between his shoulder blades that his family physician thought he had "slipped a disc." At the end of a long day of cutting hair and shaving beards, severe burning pains developed in the muscles of his back around his shoulders, and he had considerable difficulty holding his arms up to use his clippers. Even the weight of his head became unbearable when he leaned over a little to watch the movement of his scissors. When the pain was unusually severe, a dull ache radiated down both arms. After two years of traction, rest, pain pills, and learn-to-live-with-it advice, he came to me with the desperation of a man who was at the "end of the road." I instructed him to continue using moist heat, massage, and other simple physical treatments that temporarily relieved the symptoms, but I also started him on the progressive resistance exercises described in Chapter 13 (exercises 2 and 4 in particular). After two weeks, he was much improved and after six weeks, he was "cured."

Many professional men and office workers, such as dentists and accountants, work in fatiguing, static postures that result in chronic muscle pain between the shoulder blades. Most of this could be prevented with regular resistance exercise that will make the muscles more than strong enough to withstand the postural strains associated with various professions and occupations.

If you suffer from interscapular backache, be sure to read "The Muscle Inflammation of Fibromyositis" in Chapter 4.

"Crick" in the Neck (Acute Torticollis)

A telephone switch-board operator who had spent a tension-filled night after a particularly hectic day at work woke up with a sharp pain in her neck. When she turned her head to the left, she felt a jabbing pain on the left side of her neck, but she could turn her head to the right without too much difficulty. The second day her pain was worse, but on the fourth day it was almost gone.

Just about everyone has experienced the deep, sharp pain of

a "neck crick"; that is, a locking of the neck by muscle spasm. Doctors do not know much about this mysterious and aggravating disturbance, but they do have some idea of what happens to trigger the spasm.

In the greatest majority of cases, a "crick" is the result of some slight injury to fibers in a muscle that attaches to the vertebrae of the neck. The injury simply triggers the muscle into a reflex spasm that continues until the tissue products produced by the injury are absorbed or until the injury heals.

Occasionally, a "crick" is due to infection or inflammation of the involved muscles, which is sometimes secondary to throat infection. Less often, it can be the result of subluxation or slight displacement of a neck vertebra. In rare cases, spasm of the neck muscles is the result of a reflex from an organic or internal disorder.

Sudden chilling of overheated muscles, or prolonged chilling of a muscle, is a common cause of muscle inflammation and muscle spasm in the neck. Try to keep warm during and after activities that cause you to "work up a sweat," and never, under any circumstances, attempt to cool off a perspiring neck with direct cooling drafts from a fan or an air conditioner!

When a "crick" is the result of simple muscle spasm, rest and moist heat will usually take care of it in time. In most cases, however, *a muscle spasm in the neck will usually last three or four days regardless of what you do for it.* Rest should always be a part of the treatment for painful muscle spasm, and it is best to lie down and relieve the pull of gravity on the spine when the symptoms are severe. Constant tension on a muscle that is already in spasm will increase the production of irritating lactic acid (a waste product of muscular contraction) to cause further irritation in the involved muscle.

It seems that the greatest majority of "cricks" appear after a night spent in an awkward or improper sleeping position, especially after a deep or restless sleep brought on by fatigue, intoxication, or medication. Apparently, an abnormal stretch is placed upon relaxed muscle fibers, thus permitting muscle or joint injury to occur rather easily. Postural strain on the bones of the neck (as in using a pillow that is too high, or letting the head roll off a pillow that is supporting only the shoulders) can injure the joints of the neck or cause the joints to "pinch" the capsules and other soft structures that surround the joints.

Many nervous and tense persons who carry their troubles to bed with them each night will sleep with their head jammed back into their pillow from unrelieved muscle tension, so that when they awake in the morning their neck muscles are tired, stiff, and inflamed. Chapter 11, on "What to Do About Nervous Back- ache," will tell you how to get rid of your nervous tension for a good night's sleep.

Persons who suffer from chronic or recurring stiff neck can often be cured by taking muscle-strengthening neck exercises that are designed to restore the normal cervical curve. Such an exercise is described in Chapter 12 (exercise "A" of Group 11), so be sure to try it, even if you have never had a stiff neck.

Whether you are sleeping, resting, working, or playing, always try to avoid prolonged postures in which the neck must be bent or twisted. Looking up to watch parachute jumpers, for example, or looking down at a book in your lap, if continued for a long period of time, can cause acute neck pain, which may in turn cause headache or arm pain. Try to sleep and work with your neck in line with the rest of your spine. "Cricks" that are associ- ated with fever, nausea, and other symptoms of illness should be brought to the attention of a physician.

WHIPLASH—THE AUTOMOBILE NECK INJURY

Whiplash injury of the neck, which is so well known to drivers of automobiles, is, of course, an acute injury that must be treated by a doctor. When this type of injury occurs, it is usually the result of an automobile collision in which the car of the injured person is struck from behind. The sudden lurching forward of the car snaps the head of the driver backward; then, if he applies his brakes, or if his car strikes the car ahead of him, his head is again snapped forward.

The most common cause of whiplash injury is, of course, the snapping back of the head from the impact of the rear-end colli- sion. For this reason, *a head-rest piece installed just above the back portion of the seat would greatly reduce such injuries.* De- velopment of strong neck muscles would also help.

In any event, when a whiplash injury does occur, it should be treated by a doctor. Most of the time, the injury will be limited to the muscles, joints, ligaments, and soft tissues of the neck, but occasionally a vertebra will be fractured.

Disfiguring "Hump Back"—Kyphosis

Kyphosis, or "round back," is a pronounced exaggeration of the normal dorsal curve; that is, the portion of the spine between the shoulders curves sharply backward. It occurs very often in postural curvatures, as you will learn in the next chapter. But when it occurs suddenly without postural implications, it may be the result of infection or disease (such as tuberculosis or osteomalacia). When a hump-back curvature develops along with pain, fever, or illness, a thorough search should be made for disease in the thoracic vertebrae.

A postural round back looks bad enough when it occurs in men, but it is even more disfiguring in women. I once had occasion to use a very beautiful girl in illustrating a magazine article of mine on physical training, but when the photo proofs were prepared for selection, many of the photos could not be used because of the drooping appearance of a round back that had not been noticed before. Since the girl was still young, however, and since the rounded back was a postural disorder, she was completely "straightened out" by doing such postural exercises as those described in Chapter 9.

Thus, prevention of round back, especially in women, is as important for preserving physical beauty as it is for preventing backache. But prevention or correction should be started as early in life as possible.

A great many adults, especially those who are middle-aged or over, complain of becoming increasingly round shouldered in spite of exercising good posture. Assuming that these people do not have faulty posture and do not work at occupations which keep the spine bent forward, there are several possible causes of middle-aged round back.

It may not be possible to prevent some change in the normal curve of the thoracic spine when the discs and vertebrae begin to deteriorate with age, but *regular postural exercises that will strengthen the muscles of the back and the abdomen, as well as expand the chest, will aid in preventing a disfiguring round back.*

Summary

1. Because of the increased leverage placed on muscles that must hold up the spine, the shoulder girdle, and the ribs in the upper portion of the body, strong supporting muscles and good posture are especially important in preventing fatigue, pain, and disability.

2. Always try to work, sleep, and play in postures that keep your neck in line with the rest of your spine. Do not use very thick pillows under your head when you sleep on your back.

3. Try to avoid prolonged and unbroken participation in activities that call for limited movements in static postures (as in sanding a desk top or painting a ceiling). And if you feel a grating under your shoulder blades when you move your arms, do not wigwag, throw balls, paint with a roller, or do anything that increases this grating by moving your shoulder blades back and forth over your rib cage.

4. Normally, simple neck "cricks" can be treated successfully with rest and moist heat; but when they become progressively severe after three or four days, or when they are accompanied by fever and other symptoms of illness, they should be brought to the attention of your family doctor.

5. A head-rest piece installed on the back of the seat of your automobile will aid in preventing neck injuries in auto accidents.

6

General Disorders of
the Back and Spine

So far, we have considered only those disorders that occur primarily in one portion of the spine or the other. In this chapter, we will consider disorders that affect the spine as a whole. Spinal curvatures, for example, which are a common cause of low backache, are also a common cause of upper backache.

There are also some very common diseases of the vertebrae—such as arthritis and osteoporosis—that can be a cause of backache and disability anywhere in the spine. Both coping with and prevention of these disorders will be discussed in detail.

Types of Spinal Curvatures

Basically, there are two types of curvatures: functional and structural.

A *functional curvature* is a temporary curvature that straightens out when the individual lies down, and it is most often the result of muscle spasm, a fallen arch, postural changes, and other sudden changes in the body mechanics. When you stand on one leg, for example, your spine will balance itself with a functional curvature.

A *structural curvature* is a permanent curvature that has been molded by bony changes in the spine, and it will persist in any position.

Most curvatures will not become any worse after 15 years of age if postural exercises are continued throughout the individual's life. And an adult who has a spinal curvature will more readily experience backache, fatigue, and other symptoms if he fails to maintain the best posture possible by keeping the supporting muscles of his spine strong and well developed. So if you have a spinal curvature, regardless of your age, the preventive measures offered in Part II of this book will be of special importance to you in relieving backache caused by a crooked spine.

Of course, structural curvatures in adults can never be completely corrected, but exercise, improved posture, manipulation, shoe lifts, and good working conditions will be important in preventing the development of symptoms. When possible, persons with spinal curvatures should be given the type of work in which they can move around a great deal with varied use of their arm and back muscles. Static postures with limited muscular activity should be avoided.

Diseases and Infections as Causes of Curvatures

Poliomyelitis and other diseases affecting the muscles or their nerve supply can result in paralytic conditions that cause spinal curvatures. There are several diseases of the vertebrae that can cause characteristic curvature of the spine. Diseases of the chest (or chest surgery in which a portion of a lung is removed) can also result in spinal curvature. In all of these cases, however, pain and disability will make the primary disturbance obvious.

The Hump Shoulders and Pot Belly of Simple Postural Curvatures

Poor posture, even when the spine is normal, can bring about curvatures in the spine as a result of exaggeration of the normal curves of the spine. Slumping of the shoulders, for example, in habitually poor posture will permit the normal thoracic curve to sag backward into a "hump." When this hump is mild it is called a "round back," but when it becomes sharp or pronounced it is called a "kyphosis." Of course, when one portion of your spine sags, other portions must bend in opposite directions in order to balance your bodyweight. Thus, the lumbar spine (low back) balances the sagging vertebral column by increasing its normal curve or bending forward into a lordotic or sway-back position which causes a "pot belly." The neck, too, in compensating, must bend considerably in the direction of its normal curve in order to balance the head over the body. Such posture presents quite an apparition in very thin or very fat persons.

You can visualize a postural curvature by picturing a large "C" as the thoracic spine, with a small "c" fixed above and below for the cervical and lumbar spine. Both small c's should face the same direction, but in the opposite direction of the large "C."

Hump-back and sway-back curvatures of the spine resulting from poor posture tend to get worse with time if no effort is made to improve the posture or to strengthen the muscles. And when allowed to exist on into adulthood, postural curvatures become somewhat permanent. It is never too late to attempt correction for relief of symptoms, however, so be sure to read Chapter 9 on "How to Build Healthy Posture."

SHOE LIFTS FOR A SHORT-LEG CURVATURE

Many curvatures, or scolioses, in which there is a bending of the spine from side to side in an "S"-shape fashion are caused by one leg being shorter than the other. When such a deficiency is discovered in very young children, complete correction may be made by building up the shoe of the short leg until the hips are level. In the case of an adult, however, it is usually not possible to make a complete correction, since bones, muscles, and ligaments have molded themselves into the body's frame in such a way as to compensate for or strengthen the deformity. A one-inch leg deficiency, for example, can rarely be corrected more than half an inch without causing serious strain. In some cases, it might not be advisable to attempt any correction at all if the individual is not experiencing pain or disability, or if the resulting curvature has stopped short of disturbing or visible deformity.

But as you learned in Chapter 1, a "short leg" can cause acute backache, and it is no respecter of status or stature. And you know from reading Chapter 3 that a spinal curvature aggravated by a short leg and a tilted pelvis can cause many strange, "referred" pains almost anywhere in the body.

For best results, the use of heel lifts should be started while the individual is still young. And once a heel lift is prescribed, it should be used permanently.

Occasionally, X-ray examination will reveal a leg deficiency with spinal curvature in the opposite direction from that usually found in such deficiencies, thus making it impossible to correct the deficiency without increasing the curvature. For this reason, *you should not attempt to use a shoe lift without a doctor's supervision.*

While full correction of a leg deficiency may be made in children under 15 years of age, it is rarely wise for an adult to lift the shoe up more than one-half of the measured deficiency. If your doctor tells you that one of your legs is an inch shorter than the other, for example, and he tells you to build up your shoe $\frac{5}{16}$ of an inch, you might be in for trouble if you sneak around with a one-inch shoe lift.

Any leg deficiency, to be considered a possible cause of back trouble or spinal curvature, must be greater than $\frac{1}{4}$ of an inch to justify attempts at correction. Although just about everyone has a "short leg," not everyone has a deficiency that is great enough to cause trouble.

ARTHRITIS AS A CAUSE OF BACKACHE

The most common disorder of the spine is arthritis, and it is one of the most common causes of backache. Basically, the term "arthritis" implies joint inflammation, but there are many kinds of arthritis, some of which cause permanent changes in the spinal column and some of which come and go without doing much damage.

Although the causes of arthritis are not known in many cases, all arthritic victims should undergo a thorough medical examination for detection and treatment of any underlying disorder (such as anemia, kidney disease, endocrine imbalance, infection, or allergy).

Infectious forms of arthritis can be caused by such diseases as gonorrhea, syphilis, tuberculosis, and other bacterial infections, but they are not too common.

Types of Arthritis

The three types of arthritis that are a common cause of backache are *osteoarthritis, rheumatoid arthritis,* and *gouty arthritis.* We will consider below only these, all of which can be relieved considerably with home-treatment methods. Although arthritis cannot be cured in the strictest sense of the word, there is a great deal you can do to help yourself and to prevent disability from backache so that you can lead a normal life.

Osteoarthritis—The Disease of Age

The least serious but the most common type of arthritis afflicting the spine is called "osteoarthritis," which is characterized by spurring and sharp bony growths around the joints and bodies of the vertebrae. It begins primarily in middle age or later, and it attacks the joints of nearly everyone over 50 years of age, causing pain in about one person out of every 20 who are afflicted.

The symptoms of a 68-year-old retired heavy-equipment operator are typical of those experienced by persons who have moderate lumbar osteoarthritis that causes trouble. When he gets up in the mornings, his lower back is always very stiff and sore. But when he moves about a little, the stiffness decreases and he feels a little better. However, if he overexercises or becomes fatigued from standing around too long or from doing too much yard work, his symptoms become more painful and he is forced to apply moist heat and to rest until the symptoms subside. If he hurts his back a little by lifting incorrectly, he must wear a lumbosacral corset in order to get around for several days after the injury. He stretches his spine at home by using pelvic traction when he feels a pain shooting down his leg, and his wife massages the muscles of his back when muscle spasm begins to develop. (All of these techniques are discussed in Chapter 7.) Thus, by using home-treatment methods, he is able to relieve his symptoms.

Although there is no known cure for osteoarthritis, the disease is sometimes known to be the result of joint injury, excessive wear and tear on the joints, or abnormal rubbing of bone against bone in defects or deformities—which means that in many cases the disease could have been prevented. A spinal curvature, for example, which develops because of an uncorrected leg deficiency, will sometimes cause the bony overgrowth of arthritis on the inside portions of the curvature where the vertebrae are being jammed together. Deterioration of the spinal discs, when combined with bad posture and old age, will result in an abnormal amount of weight and stress being placed on the joints of the vertebrae, thus causing osteoarthritis.

Spinal traction—that is, stretching the spine with weights and a harness—may be helpful in relieving the pressure of bony spurs on delicate nerves. (Chapter 7 tells you how to rig up traction if your doctor recommends it.)

Heat, massage, aspirin (taken only when necessary to relieve pain), a good all-around diet, and exercise are frequently recommended in the treatment of osteoarthritis. Exercise, of course, should not be excessive, and it should always be stopped when pain is experienced. In other words, *you need just enough exercise to keep your muscles well toned and your joints free and movable, but not so much that the arthritic joints are aggravated.* You will have to determine for yourself how much exercise you can take.

Constipation should be corrected by eating properly, by drinking plenty of water, and by taking abdominal exercises. All excess body weight should be eliminated. Properly fitted shoes that will permit the spinal column to balance vertically without strain are important. All of these subjects are discussed in detail in Chapter 7.

Osteoarthritis does not always cause trouble, depending upon how bad it is and where it is located. We will all develop a little spinal arthritis as the years pass, but we should make every effort to prevent it by maintaining good health, by preventing and correcting mechanical deformities in the spine when possible, and by avoiding postural stresses and strains on the spinal joints. *Back exercises, chest-expanding exercises, and abdominal exercises are important in the treatment of spinal arthritis if the object is to maintain an erect, flexible spine.*

How you sit, stand, and work can have a great deal to do with the development or aggravation of spinal arthritis; so be sure to study the preventive measures outlined in Part II of this book—in the interest of both treatment and prevention.

Rheumatoid Arthritis—The Disease of Young Adults

Unfortunately, rheumatoid arthritis, one of the most serious arthritic diseases of the spine, has no known cause and is very difficult to treat. In this disease, which is far less common than osteoarthritis, the afflicted joints become painfully swollen and sometimes gradually fuse together until the joints are completely stiff or "frozen." If it starts in the spine, for example, the disease may fuse the vertebral column from bottom to top, resulting in a so-called "poker spine" or "bamboo spine." Persons who develop such an advanced form of spinal rheumatoid arthritis usually walk in a slightly bent-forward position and must turn their whole body in order to look around or turn their head.

When rheumatoid arthritis begins in the lower spine, it may cause a variety of bizarre symptoms, as it did in the case of a 26-year-old electrician. He first complained of stiffness on movement, and his symptoms were relieved by rest—just the opposite from the experience of the patient with osteoarthritis. Gradually he began to experience back pain (that seemed to radiate into his chest and abdomen) that would come and go until it began to get so bad that he experienced constant muscle spasm with an increasing amount of stiffness in his spine. Only rest and moist heat would relieve his symptoms.

Since fever and other systemic symptoms accompany rheumatoid arthritis of any type, it is believed to be caused by some kind of undetected infection or systemic disorder. When the disease is mild, it may "run a course" and burn itself out before any permanent damage or stiffness occurs in the affected joints; but when the disease is severe, the symptoms may continue until the joints become stiff, deformed, or fused, which may take several years.

When symptoms of arthritis in the spine are acute, rest is important, and massage and heat may be used over the back when they do not aggravate the symptoms. (When rheumatoid arthritis is in joints other than the spine, however, you massage *around* the affected joints rather than directly over the joints.) Simple stroking massage over the muscles of the back (to stimulate circulation and to relax muscles) is adequate. *Pounding and hacking should never be used over arthritic joints, and the use of vibrators and mechanical massagers should be prohibited.*

In any kind of spinal arthritis, you will need a firm bed along with regular postural and breathing exercises to prevent deformity in severe cases. In some cases, a back brace may be necessary. In any event, an effort should be made to keep the head up, the back straight, and the chest out, especially when rheumatoid arthritis strikes the spine. This must be accomplished by active postural exercises performed by the patient, however! Passive manipulation of the spine may aggravate the disease by stirring up and spreading the inflammation. (See Chapter 9 for simple postural exercises and instructions on how to sit and stand correctly.) Once the spine begins to stiffen up in a bent-over position, it may not be possible to prevent the deformity that compels the individual to "keep his eyes on the ground."

Since there is presently no known cause or cure for rheumatoid arthritis, treatment and prevention are very much the same; that is, improving the general health with emphasis on adequate rest, a proper diet, fresh air and sunshine, as well as avoiding fatigue and emotional stress and strain.

Gouty Arthritis—The "Big-Toe Pain" in Your Back

When some of us reach middle age, the body sometimes has trouble getting rid of uric acid, which is a by-product of certain protein foods, and the accumulating uric acid salts are deposited in the joints to cause "gouty arthritis."

Although this type of arthritis most often appears in the big toe or around the foot or knee (with visible, red swelling), it can also develop in the joints of the spine. A serum uric acid test will reveal an abnormally high level of uric acid in the blood. About 98 percent of gout patients are men. Contrary to popular belief, you do not have to "live high on the hog" to develop gout; the disease develops in rich and poor alike.

"SOFTENING" OF THE VERTEBRAE

Any sudden or rapidly developing changes in the normal curves of the spine can be indicative of bone disease. There are at least three non-infectious and non-malignant diseases—that is, Kummell's disease, osteoporosis, and osteomalacia—in which the vertebrae become so soft that they sometimes collapse under the weight of the body (or the victim may become progressively shorter in height as deformity develops in his spine).

"Softening" of the vertebrae occurs mostly in older people, and it almost always causes backache. In many cases, the causes of these diseases are not known, but there are a few things you can do that may help prevent them. Did you know, for example, that your bones can get soft from lack of exercise? And did you know that you can literally wash bone-building Vitamin D right out of your intestinal tract by using mineral oil laxatives excessively?

Kummell's Disease—The Bloodless Fracture

In this disease, the vertebrae become thin and brittle and either collapse or become compressed. Many authorities believe that the disease might be caused by injury to the spine which results in a disturbance of the blood circulation to one or more vertebrae, so that the poorly nourished bone eventually becomes so fragile that it just gives way under pressure. When this happens, there may be a sudden development of "hump back" or "flat back" (depending upon the portion of the spine involved) or some other abnormal change in the shape of the back. Most of the time, the disease occurs in the thoracic spine to cause a "hump back," but it can also cause a low backache that is associated with fatigue and pain radiating down both legs. A 75-year-old woman, for example, who complained of constant aching in her lower back and legs, was found to have a paper-thin lumbar vertebra that had collapsed like a crushed egg shell, even though she had not had an accident of any kind recently.

Since Kummell's disease may be a delayed reaction to an injury that occurred years earlier, you obviously cannot always assume that a sudden development of pain and distortion in your back is always a "muscle spasm" just because you have not had an accident of any kind, especially if you are elderly.

As we grow older, we should discontinue sports and activities in which the spine is subjected to repeated jars and strains. I know a rough-riding motorcycle racer who is 60 years of age and who repeatedly has falls and accidents that injure his back. He refuses to quit racing, however, in spite of having backache for the first time in his life.

Osteoporosis—The "Sponge Candy" Bone Disease

Spinal osteoporosis is basically a deficiency of bone material in the vertebrae, so that the affected vertebrae become light and porous like sponge candy. It is not an uncommon cause of backache in women past 50, and about three out of every ten women over 50 years of age have the disease. About one-fifth of all men over 65 years of age (who have been examined by doctors) also have osteoporosis.

When the disease is in the spine, low backache is one of the first symptoms. But if the disease progresses to the point that some of the vertebrae collapse under the weight of the body, pain and disability along with back deformity and decreasing height will become more pronounced, and the patient's capacity for physical activity becomes very limited. In fact, osteoporosis ranks closely behind arthritis as a cause of physical disability among old people, especially women.

Although osteoporosis is a disorder affecting only middle-aged and elderly persons, it has several suspected causes. In women, for example, it is sometimes caused by the hormone changes of menopause, which seem to interfere with the regeneration of new bone as the old bone breaks down. In other cases, the disease is believed to be caused by simple dietary deficiency. Thus, a doctor might prescribe hormones or food supplements containing calcium, Vitamin D, and protein, depending upon the cause of the disease.

In any event, a good, all-round diet is important in preventing the development of osteoporosis. Protein, for example, is just as important in building and maintaining bones as vitamins and minerals are—and the older we become, the more important it is to make sure that we get adequate protein, calcium, and Vitamin D in a balanced diet. In fact, persons who are 40 years of age or older should *increase* their calcium intake through milk and milk products.

One of the most common causes of osteoporosis among old people, however, is simply lack of exercise! It is well known among medical men that bones will lose their strength and substance if they are placed at rest for long periods of time. Doctors who examine returning astronauts, for example, look for osteoporosis in the bones of these "weightless" men who are not able to exercise normally for several days at a time. Bones must be used to be strong, and the amount of stress placed on a bone will largely determine its strength and its composition. For this reason, regular exercise is just as important for keeping the bones strong as it is for keeping the muscles strong.

Older people who retire to a rocking chair or a bed simply do not receive the skeletal stimulation they need to create a demand for calcium in their bones, so their bones become thin and weak from lack of healthy stress.

When advanced osteoporosis does occur in the spine, a back support may be indicated, but such support should always be accompanied by massage, alternate hot and cold applications (see Chapter 7), and special exercises to improve the circulation and to maintain muscle tone.

Good posture is very important, and a proper diet is indispensable.

Osteomalacia—"Adult Rickets"

We all know that rickets in children is caused by a deficiency of calcium and Vitamin D. Although rickets is relatively rare these days, it sometimes occurs in adults when the diet is inadequate, when there are digestive or glandular disturbances, or during pregnancy. Excessive use of laxatives in propelling undigested food from the intestinal tract, or constant use of mineral oil which "washes out" oil-soluble Vitamin D, can also cause bone-softening osteomalacia. How many people do you know who go through a daily ritual of purging their intestinal tract with high-powered laxatives?

Unfortunately, the effects of osteomalacia are seen primarily in the vertebrae where the softened bones undergo compression and distortion to cause a shortening of the trunk with a humpback deformity.

When the disease is secondary to other disturbances in the body (such as thyroid or parathyroid disease), it will be necessary, of course, to correct the underlying causes. When there is simple nutritional deficiency, your doctor may prescribe vitamin, mineral, and protein supplements, along with a warning not to use laxatives or mineral oil excessively.

Nutritionists tell us that it is difficult for an adult to get enough calcium if he does not drink at least a pint of milk each day. Cheese, cabbage, beans, turnip greens, and other green leafy vegetables, however, are also fair sources of calcium.

A deficiency of Vitamin D is the most common cause of rickets; so persons who do not drink Vitamin-D-enriched milk, or who fail to get an adequate amount of exposure to sunshine each day, should add a little fish-liver oil to their diet.

BRUCELLOSIS—THE BACKACHE YOU "CATCH" FROM ANIMALS

If you are a farmer, a veterinarian, a meat packer, or a live-stock producer who comes into contact with cattle, hogs, or goats, you might wake up one of these mornings with a fever and a backache caused by bacteria you have picked up from one of these animals if you are not careful.

The disease, called "brucellosis," is rarely fatal, and almost all of those who become infected will recover without any special treatment. But the muscle, bone, and joint pain caused by the vertebrae-invading bacteria can sometimes be shortened by treatment with certain antibiotics.

Always wear rubber gloves when handling sick or dead animals (or their discharges), and make sure that all breaks in your skin are protected against possible entrance of bacteria.

Unpasteurized milk, or cheese and butter made from unpasteurized milk, is a common source of the germ that causes brucellosis.

At the present time, it is believed that about 65 percent of human brucellosis comes from hogs. In some areas, the infection rate among hog producers is estimated to be as high as 20 percent.

Summary

1. Postural curvatures, though functional in nature in the beginning, can become structural or permanent if allowed to exist too long.
2. Adults who have arthritis or spinal curvatures should take regular exercises that are designed to strengthen the back and abdominal muscles and to expand the chest in efforts to keep the spine erect and flexible.
3. Do not build up your shoe height unless your doctor pre-

scribes it. But once prescribed, a shoe lift is generally used permanently.

4. A good all-around diet (with emphasis on protein, calcium, and Vitamin D) and plenty of sunshine are important in keeping the vertebrae hard and strong.

5. People who are middle-aged or over should take regular exercise and increase their calcium intake in order to prevent their bones from becoming weak and porous.

6. Excessive use of laxatives or mineral oil can wash bone-building Vitamin D right out of your intestinal tract, thus causing "adult rickets." Check with your doctor if you think you need a laxative every day.

7. If you have spinal rheumatoid arthritis, do not use a pillow under your knees or a thick pillow under your head when you are lying on your back.

8. Rheumatoid arthritis is a very serious disease that can permanently stiffen the affected joints. Exercise and posture should be designed to keep the joints properly aligned and as flexible as possible without increasing pain and disability.

9. If you have gouty arthritis, you will have to stick to a special diet or take special drugs to prevent the accumulation of uric acid in your body, since the cause of the disease itself cannot be corrected.

7

Effective Home Remedies
for Backaches

Since most backaches are the result of simple strains (most of which are secondary to bad posture and incorrect lifting techniques), you can, of course, do a lot to prevent backache. But when backache does occur, you can benefit from simple treatment methods that you can use right in your own home. Rest, heat, massage, a firm bed, and exercise, for example, will be effective in relieving symptoms in the greatest majority of cases, and occasionally your doctor may prescribe a back support, home traction, or a change in diet, and so on. Wearing the proper shoes can have a lot to do with how well you get along if you have chronic back trouble that has postural connections.

Thus, there are many things you can do at home to relieve the discomfort of backache, and if you understand the principles underlying the use of the various home-treatment methods, you can make better use of selected treatments by altering them to suit your needs. Cold packs, for example, may be more effective than hot packs in relieving pain and shortening disability if used during the first 12 to 24 hours following certain types of muscle injuries. But you have to know the difference between the effects of heat and cold to make the right choice in some cases.

In any event, none of the simple treatments that can be used at home are harmful or potentially dangerous. You should not assume that you cannot do anything at all without a doctor's instructions, especially when it involves basic self-help techniques that should be a part of household knowledge. Simple heat, for example, when properly applied, can provide soothing relief for minor aches and pains. If you should suffer a torn muscle or a bruising injury, you can apply a cold pack immediately to cut down on bleeding, swelling, and pain. If you waited until you could see a doctor before applying such simple treatment, the symptoms of your injury would be more pronounced and more painful, and your disability would be greater. Furthermore, since treatment of chronic backache is sometimes a long, drawn-out process that must be followed at home, it is neither sensible nor practical to think that you can depend upon your doctor or a hospital for adequate treatment over a long period of time.

Most of the time, your backache will be a minor disturbance that will respond to a few days of heat and massage, and so on, and a recurrence of symptoms can be prevented by avoiding certain stresses and strains. But if you should suffer a serious back injury that results in prolonged disability, you may have to help yourself (with your doctor's blessings, of course) if you do not want to spend half your life in a doctor's office or in a hospital. Consider the case of Mr. Doe, a self-employed truck farmer whose home and business was 40 miles from the nearest hospital.

One day when Mr. Doe was loading a truck with tomatoes and watermelons, he felt something "give" in his back. He finished loading the truck, however, even though his back was "suddenly very weak." By sundown, his back was aching severely and the pain was radiating down one of his legs. He could not sleep at all that night, and he could hardly turn over in bed. When morning finally arrived, the throbbing pain in his back and leg was severe, and he listed to one side when he stood up. He sneezed when the bright light of the sun struck his eyes, and then fell to the floor when a paralyzing pain buckled his knees. Two farm hands helped him into a car and drove him to a hospital.

The doctor agreed to let Mr. Doe go home if he would rest as necessary and if he would use home traction several hours each day, wear a back support when he got out of bed, and continue the use of moist heat and massage. And he informed Mr. Doe that he would also need a little exercise to strengthen his back when the symptoms finally subsided. "You will probably recover," he said, "but it may take time and continued treatment."

Unfortunately, few doctors have the time or the inclination to instruct a patient in the details of self-help. But if you know how to use the basic home-treatment methods, you can follow your doctor's instructions and still help yourself.

This chapter will be devoted to explaining the use of self-help techniques that are designed to relieve the symptoms of backache, but remember that the methods of prevention offered in Part II of this book should also be a part of your treatment. Many suggestions for preventing backache have also been offered in conjunction with discussion of specific ailments throughout the first part of this book, so be sure to read *all* of this book if you want to prevent the development of back trouble of any kind.

REST IS ALWAYS INDICATED

When you hurt your back, it is always a good idea to begin rest immediately if continued activity is painful or uncomfortable. Of course, when a back injury is painful, there will be little doubt about your need for rest. But there will be occasions when the injury may not seem to be painful enough to warrant "time off" from the job, even though you feel a considerable amount of discomfort. Just to be on the safe side, however, you should relieve any further stress and strain on your back after an apparent injury until at least 24 hours have passed. This will prevent any additional injury to weakened back structures, and it will give you time to evaluate the seriousness of your injury. In many cases, for example, a "not-too-serious" back strain can become quite painful after the injured tissues have had time to swell or stiffen up; and the pain and swelling may be even greater if you "finished out the day" in spite of your injury.

So for a good general rule to follow in rest for back injuries, always take the rest of the day off when you suffer a back injury that results in pain or discomfort; and then continue the rest as long as the injury is painful.

Once the acuteness of the injury has passed, however, and it is apparent that the injury is not serious and that recovery is imminent, you should begin working again—lightly at first—before you become so "out of shape" that you experience backache in once more becoming accustomed to your work. Prolonged, unnecessary rest will weaken your back rather than strengthen it.

When you do need rest for your back trouble, that does not necessarily mean that you must stay in bed 24 hours a day. When you have a nerve pain in your leg that is relieved by lying down, you should, of course, lie down as much as possible. But in many other cases, you might get along better by moving around the house a little; that is, of course, if no painful reactions occur. It is possible to aggravate a backache by staying in bed too long. Be guided by how you feel in balancing bed rest with being "up and around."

Thus, while rest for a back injury usually means "time off" from the stress and strain of house chores or employment, it does not always mean lying flat on your back.

SHOULD YOU USE HOT OR COLD APPLICATIONS?

In the greatest majority of backaches resulting from simple strain, heat will relieve pain, spasm, and stiffness by stimulating the circulation and relaxing the muscles. If the application of heat should seem to aggravate your symptoms, however, you should apply a cold pack and then wait several hours before trying the heat again.

In very painful back sprains, it is usually best to apply a cold pack as soon as possible and then wait at least 12 hours before applying heat. If heat does not increase the pain after this period of waiting, it may be continued.

Since cold is more uncomfortable than heat, many persons will prefer to try heat first; but if the heat increases pain it should not be used. When both heat and cold seem to aggravate backache resulting from a sprain, wait 24 hours or longer and then try heat. When you do find that heat seems to relieve the symptoms, apply it several times a day.

When the muscles of the back have been torn, bruised, or injured by accidents or direct blows, you should always try to use a cold pack for the first 24 hours or longer, and you should wait 36 to 48 hours before applying heat of any kind. The reason for this is obvious when you understand the effects of heat and cold. When you injure a muscle bad enough to rupture its tissues and cause bleeding or swelling (which may result in black and blue discoloration), the application of heat would increase the flow of blood in the injured fibers, thus increasing the bleeding. A cold pack, on the other hand, would restrict the flow of blood by constricting the small blood vessels, which would in turn reduce bleeding and swelling.

Most of the time, your back injuries will not be so severe that you cannot use heat from the beginning; but if you do suffer a very painful back sprain, or if there is reason to believe that you may have ruptured a muscle in your back, you should start treatment with a cold pack just to be on the safe side. You should *always* use cold when there is evidence of fresh bleeding or swelling.

In any event, back strains and sprains do not result in the amount of tissue injury and bleeding that occurs in a sprained ankle or a twisted knee; so your choice between the use of heat or cold in a fresh back injury is not so crucial as it is in injuries to joints in your arms or legs. If heat seems to aggravate your symptoms, you may simply change to cold.

When cold applications are used, they should not be applied continuously for periods longer than 24 to 48 hours, since they retard healing through constriction of the blood vessels.

When the application of heat to a back injury can be used with apparent relief of symptoms, however, it may be used indefinitely to speed healing and recovery by increasing the circulation of blood.

For simple backache in which there has not been an obvious injury, you should always try heat first. But you should not apply heat over areas where there is skin disease, infection, blood-vessel disease, or "dead" spots where you cannot feel the heat.

Alternate applications of heat and cold to chronic back conditions will alternately dilate and close tiny blood vessels to provide a "physiological massage" that will draw blood into the back and then squeeze it out again, thus providing some of the effects of active exercise without actual exertion.

HOW TO APPLY HEAT

There are several ways to apply heat to your back, and it may be "dry heat" or "moist heat."

Dry heat may be applied with an infra-red heating lamp, an electric light bulb, a hot water bottle, an electric heating pad, or a hot brick or a heated sand bag wrapped in dry towels. Grandma used to place a sheet of heavy brown paper over the muscles of the back and then "iron" them with an old-fashioned clothes iron. Painting the back with layer after layer of warm melted wax is sometimes used.

Moist heat may be applied by using towels or pieces of woolen blanket that have been wrung out in hot water; by wrapping a hot water bottle in a hot, moist towel; by shining an infra-red heating lamp down onto moist towels that have been draped over the back; by placing an insulated heating pad over warm, moist towels; or by lying down in a tub of hot water. Standing under a hot shower with a thick, heavy stream of water directed against the back is a good way to get a hot-water massage. Some drug stores sell *hydrocollator packs* which contain a substance that stays hot for at least 30 minutes after it has been boiled in water.

In any method of applying heat, you should be careful not to burn yourself. And if you use a heating pad over moist towels, make doubly sure that all electrical connections are well insulated from contact with the moisture in the towels, lest you suffer an electrical shock or burn.

Plasters (like a thick mud pie) provide an excellent form of moist heat, and they may be made out of hot mud, boiled flax-seed, a mixture of mustard and flour, or Kaolin powder.

Moist Heat Is Best!

Of all the types of heat that may be applied to the back, moist heat is perhaps the most effective. And it can be applied simply by wrapping a hot water bottle (filled with hot faucet water) in a piece of woolen blanket that has been wrung out in hot water. Both the back and the bottle should then be covered with a sheet of plastic or oil cloth in order to hold in the heat. Just leave the application on until it cools off and then reapply it 3 or 4 times a day.

You should not use boiling hot water in a hot water bottle if it is to be applied to the body, since the excessive heat may penetrate the towels to cause a burn. Water that is heated to about 125 degrees Fahrenheit should be hot enough. If you think the bag is a little too hot, wrap it in two towels and then remove one of the towels when the bottle begins to cool off.

In order to make sure that a hot water bottle is not too stiff to fit itself to the contours of the body, partially fill it with water and then squeeze the bag until the water comes to the top before you screw in the stopper. This will remove all of the air from the bottle and prevent overfilling.

Although water as hot as 135 degrees Fahrenheit is sometimes used in hot water bottles that are wrapped in towels, water hotter than 115 degrees should not be allowed to come into direct contact with the skin, since a burn could result. When using mud packs or melted paraffin in applying heat to the body, however, temperatures of 120 to 125 degrees can be used because the specific heat of these substances is lower than that of water. For example, water heated to 130 degrees would burn or blister the skin, whereas mud or paraffin heated to the same temperature could be tolerated.

If you are not sure about the temperature of a hot application, always test it by touching it to the inside of your forearm before placing it on the body.

When you are using a heat lamp to keep moist towels hot over the back, the distance of the lamp from the towels will vary from 12 to 24 inches, depending upon the size of the lamp. If you are not sure about the distance, place the lamp well above the towels and then gradually move it down until a comfortable heat is felt.

Most hot applications should last from 15 to 30 minutes. At the conclusion of each application, cover the back with a piece of warm flannel in order to prevent chilling.

If your back is sore and stiff when you get up in the morning, apply a little heat before you begin the day. You will find that it will loosen up your back considerably.

When moist applications of any kind are used several times during the day, it is always a good idea to rub a little baby oil into the skin after each application in order to prevent the skin from "drying out" or becoming chapped.

When massage is used, it should be applied *after* the heat has been applied. In the next few pages, you will find a simplified back-massaging technique that anyone can use.

Do not substitute dry heat for moist heat unless you have to. Moist heat has a much more pronounced effect on blood circulation, since it reflexly dilates the deeper-lying blood vessels; and it is more effective in relieving pain and relaxing muscles. Much of the dry heat you use is dissipated by the circulation of blood just beneath the skin.

Warning: If you have diabetes, ask your doctor about the safety of the type of heat you are using.

Painting the Spine With Paraffin

Persons who do not want to use moist heat applications or a dry heating pad might want to try painting a sore or arthritic portion of the back with melted paraffin. This form of heat treatment is less messy than plasters (though it may be less effective than simple moist heat) and less trouble than using hot bricks or sand bags wrapped in towels. And it may be more effective than a dry heating pad. Furthermore, the same paraffin can be used over and over.

Go to the grocery store and buy about 4 pounds of ordinary commercial paraffin and a pound of light mineral oil. Mix the paraffin and oil by heating and stirring it in a big double boiler until all of the paraffin has melted. (When you want to mix smaller amounts, mix one part mineral oil to 4 parts paraffin.) The mixture should not be hotter than 125 degrees when it is applied to the skin. If you do not have a thermometer to test the temperature of the paraffin, just remove it from the stove and let it cool until the surface begins to congeal before you use it.

Use a soft paint brush that is about 2 inches wide or wider and "paint" the back with the paraffin until a cast about one-half inch thick has been formed. It will take several layers, of course, to form a coat this thick—and the application should be applied only over the portion of the back causing trouble.

After you have applied an adequate amount of paraffin, place a sheet of wax paper over the application and then cover it with a piece of flannel in order to keep the paraffin from cooling off too rapidly. Leave the application on for 30 minutes or longer.

After the paraffin has cooled off, or when the treatment is discontinued, just peel the paraffin off the skin and save it for the next application.

The first coating of paraffin will, of course, feel pretty hot. But excessive heat will not be felt on subsequent coatings. In any event, the second or two of intense heat felt when the paraffin is applied accounts for its effectiveness in relieving soreness.

The best position for applying hot paraffin to the back is the face-down position, but a pillow may have to be placed under the pelvis to lessen strain on the lower back.

If the patient has to lie on his side for this treatment, wrap a piece of wide gauze around his body so that the first coat of paraffin can anchor itself in the gauze to avoid slipping from the skin.

Caution: Paraffin is inflammable, so be careful not to spill any over an open flame. And be sure to shave hairy backs before applying the paraffin!

How to Make a Poultice

A poultice supplies a good form of moist heat, and it seals off the treated area for an even and constant distribution of heat.

Flaxseed (linseed) is the most popular ingredient of heat plasters, and it will retain heat for a considerable period of time. Here is how you can make a *flaxseed poultice:*

Mix 1 cup of flaxseed with 1½ cups of water and boil it until it is thick and mushy like bread dough. Then take the mixture off the stove and beat it up with a half teaspoon of sodium bicarbonate.

Spread the mixture about one inch thick over a piece of muslin that has been spread out in a bread pan that is being kept warm by the eye of a stove. Place another sheet of muslin over the top of the spread mixture and fold the ends over to prevent leakage. Be sure to cut the muslin to the correct size beforehand so that the poultice will not be too large when you place it over the back.

You can keep the poultice in place during side-posture treatment by tying it to the back with a wide strip of muslin that will reach around the body.

Leave the application on the back until it cools off; it should be good for at least 30 minutes.

When the poultice is removed, wash the skin with soap and warm water, and then rub the skin with baby oil or petrolatum (petroleum jelly) in order to prevent dryness of the skin. Avoid chilling by covering the treated area with a piece of warm flannel.

Since it is always a good idea to follow heat with a little massage, you can take advantage of the oil rub by massaging the muscles of the back.

When you have finished with the pot in which you boiled the flaxseed, fill it up with cold water so that it will be easier to clean later or you will have a major pot-cleaning chore awaiting you.

Mustard Plasters for Arthritis

If you have chronic back arthritis, any of the forms of heat discussed so far may be effective in relieving the soreness, but you might find that a mustard plaster will be more effective in relieving the pain. In addition to the heat supplied by such a plaster, the skin-irritating oil of the mustard acts as a "counter-irritant" which may reflexly relieve the pain in the joints. It is believed, for example, that the harmless irritation produced on the skin by the volatile mustard oil will release a histamine-like substance through the nerves to soothe inflammation deep within the joints. In any event, here is your formula for making a *mustard plaster:*

Mix 1 part dry mustard with 4 to 6 parts flour for adults (12 parts flour to 1 part mustard for children), and then stir in just enough warm water to make a smooth paste. *Do not boil the mixture, and do not use hot water!* If the temperature of the water you use is over 140 degrees Fahrenheit, the oil of the mustard will not be released and the plaster will not be effective.

Spread the mustard paste about one-quarter of an inch thick over a sheet of muslin, and then prepare the plaster in the same way you prepare a flaxseed poultice.

When the plaster has been applied to the back, lift up the plaster and examine the skin every 5 minutes for redness. After 5 to

20 minutes, the skin should begin to get a little pink. *When a definite pink color appears, remove the plaster.* Severe blistering can result if you leave the plaster on too long!

When the plaster is removed, wash the skin with soap and warm water and apply oil to prevent the skin from chapping.

WHEN YOU NEED A COLD PACK

If you cannot tolerate heat, or if you should suffer a painful injury, you may find a cold application more effective in relieving your pain. Almost any painful condition can be relieved to some extent by the numbing effects of cold, but since heat is more effective in promoting healing, cold is not usually used longer than 48 hours—and then only if there is acute inflammation or swelling.

There are some people, however, who cannot tolerate heat of any kind; for them, cold may be more effective if used occasionally to relieve pain and muscle spasm. (There are also a few people who are "allergic" to cold.)

Cold applications may be made by wringing towels out in ice water; by making a compress out of ice cubes, a plastic bag, and a moist towel; or by filling an ice coil, an ice bag, or a hot water bottle with crushed ice. Ice should never be applied directly to the skin, since it could damage the body tissues.

Leave the application on for about 20 or 30 minutes if no discomfort occurs. Repeat the application several times a day.

Doctors sometimes use ethyl chloride spray to chill an injured muscle (and to relax muscle spasm) until an ice pack can be applied. Coaches and athletes who need cold applications in an emergency for treatment of athletic injuries often use chemically treated "ice bags" that get cold when they are broken open. In severe injuries in which there is black and blue discoloration, cold should be applied continuously for the first day or so.

Quick Cold at Home

If you have no special equipment at home for making a cold pack, you can easily make one by filling a hot water bottle with crushed ice and applying it directly to the skin. A small, moist towel wrapped once around the bag will prevent a biting chill.

If you have no crushed ice for use in a regular ice bag, you can partially fill a plastic bag with ice cubes and water so that the bag can mold itself to the contours of the back. Apply the bag over a moist cloth that has been laid over the back, and then cover both the bag and the back with a sheet of oil cloth or plastic to hold in the cold.

Alternating Heat and Cold

If you want to try alternating hot and cold applications on your back to "flush out" healing muscle injuries or to increase the circulation of blood through osteoporotic vertebrae (see Chapter 6), you will need two rubber or plastic containers, one filled with hot tap water and one filled with crushed ice or ice cubes.

Start off by using the heat. Apply the heat for about 15 minutes and the cold for about 5 minutes. Precede the application of heat with a hot, moist towel laid over the back, and then lay the hot water bottle over the towel. Precede the application of cold with a cold towel over the back in the same manner. Cover the applications with a rain coat or a sheet of plastic or oil cloth to prevent the circulation of air.

Alternate the hot and cold applications two or three times, and make sure that you end up with the heat.

You may have to refill the hot water bottle between applications in order to keep it hot, but the ice bag should last for the duration of the treatment.

If you simply want to wring towels out in hot water and cold water for alternating heat and cold (contrast bathing), your cold water should be 55 degrees Fahrenheit or lower, and your hot water should not be hotter than 125 degrees.

A Simple Technique for Massaging the Back

After rest and heat, massage is the next most important home-treatment for backache. Just about everyone, at one time or another, has been called upon to massage the aching back of some member of the family. And as you learned earlier, massage is a very valuable addition to the application of heat.

Since massage is a treatment that should be applied daily over a long period of time for best results, it would be foolish and expensive to visit a physical therapist or a doctor for such simple treatment.

Unfortunately, many people think that massage should be a complicated technique that must include all sorts of pounding, pulling, and probing to be effective. This is not true, especially in the case of the muscles of the back. In fact, few people who have an acute backache can tolerate the hacking and pounding of an athlete's rubdown, and such jarring massage can greatly aggravate an arthritic spine. All that is really needed is a good firm stroking or kneading that follows the course of the big muscles that travel along each side of the spinal column.

When you are massaging someone's back, always have him lie down so that the blood circulation will not have to flow uphill in its journey back to the heart; and then rub toward the head so that the pressure you place on the muscles will push the venous blood toward the heart.

Here is a simple technique that anyone can follow:

Start at the bottom of the spine near the hips. Place one hand on each side of the spine, with the thumbs over the center of the back and the closed fingers slanted off on each side so that the hands are molded to the ridges of muscle that run parallel to the spine.

Then, with a firm pressure, stroke slowly and smoothly toward the head, moving both hands together about 5 or 6 inches up the back. Finish each stroke by sliding the hands off to the side so that the thumbs move over and across the ridges of muscle. Overlap your strokes until you have covered the entire length of the spine. Massage the back about 3 times.

In order to prevent excessive irritation and friction on the skin, and to facilitate the actual massage, use a small amount of lubricant, such as baby oil or Dermassage. When the massage is completed, a little rubbing alcohol can be used to remove the oil.

If you use alcohol at home, do not use this very inflammable substance near a heating lamp or an open flame. I know of an instance in which someone tried splashing alcohol over his back while he was under a carbon-arc type of heat lamp. Somehow a spark ignited the alcohol, and before he could think to roll over on his back and smother the flames, he suffered a bad burn.

In addition to providing pure pleasure, massage opens up many normally closed capillaries (small blood vessels), stimulates circulation, relaxes muscles, and promotes healing.

If you should suffer a severely torn back muscle, however, massage should not be used until the injured fibers have knitted together enough to withstand pressure and stretching. In serious injuries of this type, your doctor will provide you with adequate instructions. In any event, since massage should not be painful, you can be guided by the absence or presence of pain in applying massage for any condition.

Massage With a Vibrator

Persons who do not have a painful spinal arthritis or a torn back muscle and who want a good stimulating massage may combine stroking movements with the application of a small hand vibrator. When possible, use a rubber, suction-cup tip on the vibrator (sold in any drug store).

With the vibrator in one hand, and the other hand placed over the ridge of back muscles on one side of the spine, lock the tip of the vibrator up under the thumb and first finger of the massaging hand (with the hand and the vibrator tip flattened against the back); then move the hand and the vibrator as a unit up the back. Use a lubricant with short stroking movements as in regular massage—and massage both sides of the back. Of all the types of massage I have tried on the backs of patients, this massage-with-a-vibrator technique has been the most effective and the most well-received.

Remember that massage should never be painful, so always keep it light enough to be comfortable. An excessive amount of stimulating massage in elderly or physically unfit persons may result in fatigue and mild fever from a "systemic poisoning" caused by the "flushing out" of waste products, stagnant tissue fluids, and debris that have accumulated in injured or unused muscles. So begin lightly and increase the amount of massage applied over a period of several days. Ten or 15 minutes of massage will be enough for most persons when the entire back is covered.

When massage is applied lightly with only the hands, it is very relaxing and tends to promote sleep; but when it is applied vigorously or with a vibrator, it is physically stimulating.

A FIRM MATTRESS IS IMPORTANT

Everybody should sleep on a firm mattress, especially those who have back trouble. When you go to bed for a good night's sleep, the muscles in your back relax and the ligaments of the spine must assume most of the responsibility for holding the vertebrae in correct alignment. Obviously, if the bed sags excessively, a considerable amount of strain would be placed on the joints and ligaments of the spine—and this could greatly aggravate backache.

If your mattress seems to sag too much, that is, if your body does not rest in a position in which all portions of your spine are in correct alignment, a board (preferably a one-half-inch-thick sheet of plywood that has been cut to the same length and width as the mattress) placed between the mattress and the springs will firm up your bed. (You may hinge the board in the middle for convenience in transferring it from one bed to another if you travel. Many hotels furnish bed boards on request.)

A simple cotton, felt, or hair-stuffed mattress, if evenly packed, would be best in most cases. Inner spring mattresses are sometimes satisfactory if the springs can mold themselves to the contours of the body and still support the spine in a level, horizontal position.

It is, of course, possible to make a mattress too hard, especially when there is acute back pain. No mattress should be so hard or so thin that it cannot mold itself to the normal curves of the spine. Some persons may even find that a board under the mattress is uncomfortable in the first stages of a severe back injury, and they may have to wait a few days before inserting the board permanently.

In any event, persons who have chronic back trouble should probably use a bed board for the rest of their lives; and, as I said earlier, everybody should have a firm mattress. But do not be like the patient who aggravated his back trouble by sleeping on a hardwood floor because his doctor had advised him to "sleep on a board." I know of several instances in which patients literally slept on a board because they failed to understand that the board was to be inserted between the mattress and the springs.

AN EXTRA PILLOW IN BED IS USEFUL

Even when a good, firm mattress is used, it may be necessary, in many cases, for persons with back trouble to provide special support for their arms or legs in order to rest comfortably. When you sleep on your back, for example, there is normally a slight arching up of the lower back when the legs are lying flat on the mattress—and this could aggravate almost any kind of low-back trouble. For this reason, *a pillow should be placed under both knees so that they can rest in a slightly bent or flexed position when a patient who has a low-back strain is lying on his back,* thus relieving the tension on the lumbar spine. (Persons who have rheumatoid arthritis, however, should not use a pillow under their knees, since this might produce stiff, bent knees or a rounded back. See "Rheumatoid Arthritis—The Disease of Young Adults" in Chapter 6.) See Figure 2 for pillow placement.

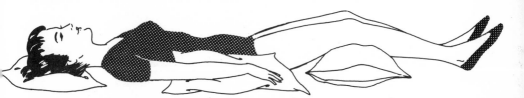

**Figure 2: Placement of extra pillows
for additional support and comfort**

Although "stomach sleeping" should be avoided most of the time, it can sometimes be done comfortably (especially during the application of heat and massage) by placing a pillow under the pelvis so that the spine will be arched up slightly. (Since the joints of the spine are on the back side of the vertebral column, prolonged "back bending" by sleeping in an unsupported face-down position, especially on a soft mattress, can jam the vertebral joints together and result in a painful stiffness in the spine, even when the spine is normal.)

Sleeping on your side in certain types of back trouble can be accomplished more comfortably by placing a pillow between slightly bent knees. And persons who have large hips and a small waist must sometimes place a thin pillow between their waist and the mattress in order to keep their spine from sagging down when lying on their side.

As a general rule, no head pillow should be used when sleeping face down, and only a thin pillow—or no pillow at all—should be used when sleeping on your back. However, a fairly thick pillow should be used under your head when you are lying on your side.

In any event, if you have back trouble, you may find that an extra pillow in bed can be very useful for providing additional support in certain sleeping postures. Be sure to read "How to Have a Healthy Posture Lying Down" in Chapter 9.

DON'T FORGET TO EXERCISE!

Once you have overcome the pain and disability of acute backache by using rest, heat, and massage, you should begin to take a little light exercise as soon as possible. When a muscle has been injured, the involved fibers sometimes become "glued" together by escaped tissue fluids and by scar tissue if they are not adequately exercised soon enough. Also, an injured joint that has been placed at rest too long may become stiff and chronically "sore" from adhesions that have formed between and around the joint surfaces.

Obviously, a little movement should be started as soon as freedom from pain will permit if the joint surfaces and the individual muscle fibers are to remain free and movable as healing takes place. (Normally, each muscle fiber moves separately, but when adhesions form from lack of exercise following an injury, the damaged muscle fibers become stuck together like a stack of wet stamps.)

To begin with, however, the exercise should not be too heavy or too vigorous, and movements should be limited to a little bending and stretching—such as bending the trunk lightly in all directions. Then, when the back seems to be getting back to normal, the exercises described in Chapter 12 can be started in order to strengthen the supporting muscles of the spine.

Orthopedists tell us that weak muscles alone are a common cause of backache, and that they contribute greatly to back injury; so when your back has been injured, it is doubly important to strengthen your back muscles to prevent easy recurrence of the injury.

Persons who fail to follow-up recovery with exercise are very likely to have back trouble again. And the more often back trouble occurs, the more likely it is to become chronic or permanent.

If you should suffer a slipped disc, a ruptured back muscle, or a severe ligamentous strain, all of which are painful injuries that will compel you to see a doctor, recovery prior to exercise will take a little longer than if you suffered a simple back strain, but you can be guided by how you feel and by your doctor's instructions in performing your exercise. Do not do any exercise that seems to hurt your back or cause a recurrence of symptoms.

The free-hand exercises described in Chapter 12 are adequate for strengthening the muscles that support the spine, but progressive resistance exercises such as those described in Chapter 13 are best for building overall, extraordinary body strength that will protect the spine during heavy exertion or during physical emergencies.

How to Wear a Back Support

Unless you should suffer a "slipped disc" or a bad sacroiliac strain, it is not very likely that you will ever need to wear a back support, since most back strains will "get well" with rest, heat, massage, and exercise. But there may be occasions when a support will be helpful in permitting you to return to work a little sooner than usual in filling an important position or in earning a badly needed paycheck. Except in rare cases, however, the use of a back support is just a temporary measure, and it should be discarded as soon as possible. Even in bad back injuries, back supports should not be worn too long after back pain has disappeared, since the muscle weakness resulting from prolonged support will break down the muscle guard needed to protect the spine during physical effort.

When you do wear a back support for a considerable period of time, you should begin your exercises *before* the support is discarded. The support should simply be removed once or twice a day for the exercises and then slipped back on during hours of employment; then, when the time comes to discard the support, well-developed muscles can take over the job of holding the spine erect.

I knew a 34-year-old construction worker who wore a heavy steel brace so long that he felt that he could not get along without it, even though his back was no longer painful. And everytime he tried working without his brace, he hurt his back in carrying out routine job assignments. So rather than have him discard his brace all at once, I suggested that he begin taking exercises such as those in Chapters 12 and 13, and then gradually discard the brace—beginning with a few hours each morning before his muscles became fatigued—until he could go without it completely. In this way, he eventually made a full recovery and was able to work full time without the brace.

Back supports are seldom used in the treatment of muscular injuries, although they are sometimes used in supporting injured joints and ligaments when an individual chooses to go back to work before the injury has healed adequately.

In any event, most back supports are prescribed for disc injuries and ligamentous strains which require long periods of rest and inactivity for recovery. And the muscle weakness that usually results from such injuries must be overcome by exercises that are designed to strengthen the muscles without straining the joints, discs, or ligaments.

Muscle injuries, of course, can very often be treated from the beginning with light exercise, but injured ligaments must be treated with complete rest so that they will have ample time to heal and tighten up before heavy work is resumed. Ligaments that are strained repeatedly become stretched and relaxed, resulting in a "loose" joint that is subject to recurring strains. This is why a support is sometimes recommended in bad back strains, and why exercise that has been designed to strengthen the supporting muscles should be started before the support is discarded.

Since most back supports should be removed for daily heat, massage, exercise, and other forms of physical treatment, it is rarely practical to tape the back with adhesive strapping. Tape provides very little support for the spine, and it is difficult to apply and remove. Applied over one side of the body, tape simply rides the skin over the muscles (shutting out the air and sealing off the pores), and it sometimes causes a very annoying skin irritation. Effective support for the spine can be accomplished only by encircling the trunk with a semi-rigid corset. So if your doctor does not "tape your back up" like the doctor down the street, that does not necessarily mean that he is not treating you properly.

Most people prefer to wear their back supports over their underwear so that the support will not become soaked with perspiration. When a heavy-duty, canvas-like support is worn next to the body, talcum powder applied between the skin and the support will help prevent excessive rubbing.

Back supports are, of course, also prescribed for fractures, spinal tuberculosis, and other serious disturbances of the spine. In these cases, complete rest is usually imperative, and exercise may be started only on approval of the attending physician.

In the greatest majority of cases, a ready-made support properly fitted by a surgical supply house will provide adequate support for your back. In the more serious type of back injury, however, it may be necessary for an orthopedic specialist to prescribe a made-to-order steel brace from an orthopedic brace shop.

In any event, let your doctor prescribe the type of support you need. A low-back injury, for example, might call for a wide *lumbosacral support* which splints the entire lumbar spine, whereas a sacroiliac strain would call for a narrow, strap-like *sacroiliac belt*. Severe neck injuries usually call for a *cervical collar*.

If you should go by a drug store and ask for a "back support," you will probably be given a sacroiliac belt. And if your neighbor offers to loan you a back support, it might be the wrong size in the wrong support for the wrong condition. So do not wear a support unless you need one—and then let your doctor tell you what you need.

HOW TO RIG UP TRACTION AT HOME

When you have an arm or leg pain that is being caused by a nerve being pinched or irritated somewhere in your vertebral column, your doctor might prescribe spinal traction. When properly applied, traction will pull the vertebrae apart and relieve the pressure on joints and discs, thus, in many cases, removing the pressure on spinal nerves.

Most physicians hospitalize patients who need spinal traction, but this kind of treatment can also be given in the home. Surgical and orthopedic supply houses will usually rent the necessary equipment on a doctor's orders for a surprisingly small weekly charge. Since the treatment for a "slipped disc" or an arthritic condition (in which spurs are pressing upon nerves) is usually long and drawn out, home traction is sometimes more practical than hospital traction when there are no complications.

Traction may be applied from either end of the spine, depending upon the portion of the spine involved. A disc injury or a "pinched nerve" in the neck, for example, would be treated with cervical traction, whereas a low-back condition would be treated with pelvic or lumbar traction. Some doctors recommend ankle traction (that is, the traction pulls from the ankles) in low-back disorders, but I have never been able to see how such treatment could effectively stretch the spine.

In any event, your doctor will prescribe the type of traction you need, and, if you choose to use such treatment in your home, an orthopedic supply house will install the equipment for you and supply you with the correct amount of weight. Many persons are able to make their own traction equipment after they have seen it used.

Spinal traction is usually safe and harmless as described here, and it may be used without a doctor in constant attendance. When used at home, however, each application of traction, which may last from 15 minutes to several hours, should be terminated when discomfort arises from fatigue or pain. When spinal traction is indicated, it should provide some immediate relief from pain.

Cervical Traction—"Stretching Your Neck"

Traction on the neck is best applied in a position in which the individual is lying flat on his back for greater muscular relaxation, although it may also be applied in a sitting position in a doorway. See Figure 3 for neck or cervical traction.

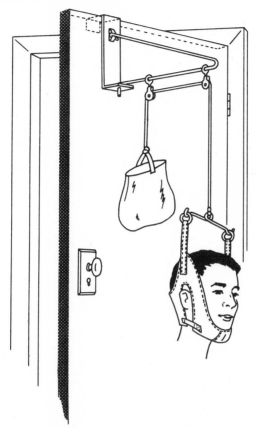

Figure 3: Cervical traction

For traction while lying down, attach one end of a heavy cord to a harness that will pull against the base of the skull and the bottom of the chin. Pass the other end of the cord over a pulley that is attached to the head of the bed (or to a wall), and then attach a weight (5 to 15 pounds—a bag of sand, for example) to the dangling end of the cord. Make sure that the pulley is on a level with the head so that the traction will stretch the spine through its central axis.

Five to ten pounds of weight will be sufficient for traction over a long period of time (an hour or more); up to 15 pounds may be used for shorter periods of time. Just select a weight that gives you a comfortable and painless traction. Too heavy a weight will cause your neck muscles to tense up in resistance, thus nullifying the effects of the traction. Ask your doctor before using heavier weights.

Some people delight in saying that their doctor "hangs" them when he applies neck traction, and such careless statements frighten some people into believing that such treatment is painful. When properly applied, however, traction is relaxing and comfortable.

Lumbar (Pelvic) Traction—Stretching Your Lower Back

Pelvic traction for the lumbar spine is usually applied by using a pelvic harness that is attached to cords which pass over pulleys fastened to the foot of the bed. One type of harness has a cord attached on each side of the harness (both cords attached to a "foot board" from which a single cord passes over a pulley), and another type has a single cord attached to a flap on the back of the harness.

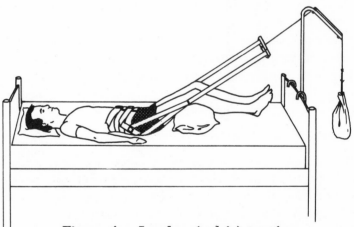

Figure 4: Lumbar (pelvic) traction

The harness with the single cord and the back flap is probably the most effective, since the flap projects down to provide a "slide" for the buttocks so that the pull from the cord passing up between the legs will flatten the lumbar spine by lifting the pelvis during traction.

Fifteen to 30 pounds of weight are usually used in pelvic traction, depending upon the tolerance and the condition of the individual. As a general rule, traction on the lumbar spine should be applied an hour or two at a time, several times a day, or as often and as long as needed to relieve pain in the legs. Traction is rarely used or needed when there is no radiating nerve pain.

In most cases, the foot of the bed should be elevated several inches so that a counter traction will make up for the loss of traction brought about by the buttocks dragging against the mattress. A brick—or two bricks—under each foot post would do fine. And it would be helpful to occasionally reach back over your head and pull your body back toward the head of the bed while the traction is being applied.

Most pelvic traction should be rigged up to pull at an angle of 30 degrees or so, thus lifting the pelvis from the bed in order to lessen drag and to flex the spine slightly (so that the openings on the back of the spine where the nerves are passing through will be larger). Placing a pillow under both knees will help. (The angle of the traction cord should be just high enough to permit the cord to pass *over* the pillows.)

Traction machines, in which traction is applied horizontally by springs or motors, offer an effective form of traction when the upper body is strapped down while the lower spine is being stretched. But this type of traction is usually available only in doctors' offices or in hospitals.

Traction With a Chair

If you have low backache and a slight leg pain, and you are "too busy" or in too much of a hurry to bother with pelvic traction, you can get a little traction by lying down on the floor with your legs up on a chair in the following manner:

Lie on your back on a rug-covered floor and place your lower legs over the arms of a large padded chair or sofa. You should actually be in a sitting position while lying down, with your trunk, thighs, and legs at right angles to each other; and the chair supporting your legs (from the knees down) should be just high enough that your hips are lifted from the floor slightly. You may have to place a couple of cushions between your legs and the supporting chair arm to get the lift you need. Lie relaxed in this position for three or four minutes. (See Figure 5.)

Since the joints of the spine, and the openings through which the spinal nerves pass, are on the back side of the vertebral column, the lifting effect provided by the support of the chair will round-out the lumbar spine and open up the bony rings containing the nerves, thus relieving nerve and joint pressure.

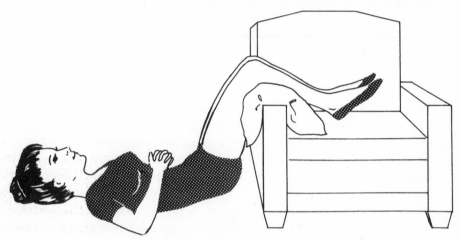

Figure 5:   Traction with a chair

Lying on your side and pulling your bent knees up toward your chest might also be of value in relieving backache and leg pain, especially if you are sway-backed.

Hanging from a doorway chinning bar several times a day is a good way to relieve pressure on joints and discs. Supporting your weight on stiff arms between two chairs that have been turned back to back will provide fairly good low-back traction if you can learn to relax the muscles in your lower back.

It will take a little practice to suspend your bodyweight on stiff arms while relaxing the muscles of your back, however, and to do this you will have to let both feet rest on the floor in a relaxed manner. But once you get the knack of it, you will be able to feel your lumbar spine stretch under the weight of your lower body. Your body and your arms should be vertical, of course, and you should be in the same position you would be in if you were about to do "dips" between two chair backs.

Good Foot Posture and Proper Shoes Are Important

Your feet and your shoes are also important factors to be considered in the cause and cure of your backache. It is well known, for example, that a rolling-in of the ankles (resulting from bad foot posture, weak ankles, or worn shoes) will cause an inward rotation of the thighs and legs, which, in turn, will transmit a strain to the knees and the lower back to cause a sway back.

Shoes with heels that are too high will also place considerable strain on the lower back by tilting the pelvis forward and causing a sway-back condition, which may result in a compensatory "round back" in the upper spine.

Occasionally, shoes without heels will result in a "flat-back" backache that is caused by the pull of abnormally short and tight hamstrings (muscles and tendons on the back of the legs). Women, for example, who have worn high-heeled shoes so long that structural changes (shortening) have taken place in their leg tendons, sometimes experience backache when they suddenly change to low-heeled shoes. (See "Stretching Tight Ankle Tendons" in Group 9 of Chapter 12.)

Fallen arches, bunions, foot injuries, and other disturbances of the feet, as well as improperly fitted or worn-out shoes, can cause backache by throwing the spine out of balance. If you have foot trouble of any kind, you should have it taken care of whether you now have backache or not. If your family doctor cannot handle your foot problems, he can recommend a good chiropodist or an orthopedic specialist.

Make sure that your shoes are one-quarter to one-half inch longer than your feet, and wide enough to accommodate your feet without squeezing them. It is important that your shoes be made to fit your feet rather than force your feet to fit your shoes. Select a good leather shoe that has a thick sole and a rigid shank; that is, the arch of the shoe between the front sole and the heel should not bend very easily.

The rubber and cloth type of shoe that rolls or gives under pressure will not give your feet any support at all, especially if you have a job in which you must do a great deal of standing or walking. Unless you already have fallen arches, however, you should not buy shoes that have built-in arch supports.

Exercises designed to strengthen the feet and ankles (such as the "Toe Rises With a Barbell," exercise 10 in Chapter 13) are important in maintaining good foot posture for good back posture.

Try to avoid walking "slue-footed" (toes pointed out) or "pigeon-toed" (toes pointed in); keep your toes pointed fairly straight ahead.

If you do not think your feet can make your back ache, then consider this case history: Mrs. B.C., age 44, had a ten-year history of chronic backache with leg pain. She had seen a number of doctors in seeking a cure for her condition, but nothing helped (including exercises). One doctor told her that she had a "disc protrusion" and recommended surgery. Physical and X-ray examination revealed that she was extremely sway-backed and that her bad posture was being aggravated by a rolling in of both ankles. When her foot posture was corrected with laced-up oxfords that had built-in sole wedges, her back straightened up enough to relieve the pressure on joints and nerves; and after 6 weeks of postural exercises while wearing the corrective shoes, her backache disappeared.

Thus, in many cases, good foot posture is just as important as good spinal posture in preventing backache. "How to Assume Good Standing and Walking Posture" in Chapter 9 will tell you more about building good foot posture.

Don't Take Too Many Vitamins!

If you take vitamins for "preventive medicine," or if your doctor prescribes Vitamins A or D, etc., do not take any more than the label on the bottle suggests. An excessive amount of these vitamins in a high-powered formula can cause bone changes in your vertebral column from *hypervitaminosis*, which may result in backache along with other symptoms of illness.

The Backache of Constipation

Constipation, the "great American disease," causes backache by overloading the colon. This highly distressing condition can be prevented by drinking plenty of water, by eating foods that contain roughage (such as fruits and whole grain cereals and breads), and by making sure that you have regular toilet hours.

Many busy people who have too much to do each day will sometimes postpone toilet functions for 24 hours or longer. As a result, the colon absorbs the water from the accumulating waste matter, leaving the contents of the colon hard, impacted, and greatly enlarged. In these cases, an enema is needed to break up the impactions, thus cutting a pattern for chronic constipation.

Excessive use of laxatives to promote bowel activity by irritating the intestinal tract can, of course, result in chronic constipation, since the bowels become "addicted" to the laxative stimulation. There are many people who eat concentrated and refined foods all day and who then take a laxative each night or an enema each morning in an effort to get rid of the sticky residue in their bowels. You can be spared from such a depressing fate if you will exercise a little informed caution on the side of prevention.

Regular abdominal or situp exercises (such as those in Group 3 of Chapter 12) might be helpful in keeping the intestinal tract loose and active.

Summary

1. If you should hurt your back on the job, take the remainder of the day off if you experience a considerable amount of discomfort, and then continue the rest from day to day as long as the injury is painful. Rest is always indicated in painful back injuries.
2. Cold packs should be used during the first 36 to 48 hours in severe injuries in which there is a great deal of pain, swelling, bleeding, or tearing of tissues.
3. Most minor back injuries will respond to heat, but when heat seems to aggravate symptoms, apply a cold pack and wait 24 to 36 hours before trying heat again.
4. Moist heat is better than dry heat! A hot water bottle filled with hot faucet water and wrapped in a moist towel is a simple and effective way to apply heat.
5. If you have spinal arthritis, try the mustard plaster described in this chapter.
6. Light, comfortable massage following hot applications should be applied over oiled skin in a stroking movement toward the heart.

7. A firm mattress is important in treatment and prevention of backache, but the mattress should not be so hard that it cannot mold itself to the normal curves of the spine. A thick sheet of plywood between your mattress and your springs will firm up your bed.

8. If you do not have rheumatoid arthritis in your spine, a pillow placed under both knees while you are lying flat on your back can be used to relieve back pain caused by strain or injury.

9. Light muscle contraction and joint movement for maintaining flexibility should be started (after an injury) as soon as freedom from pain will permit. Then, in order to strengthen the back muscles for preventing recurrence of back injury, progressive resistance exercise should be taken.

10. If you wear a back support that has been prescribed by your doctor, you should begin your back-strengthening exercises *before* you discard your support for good.

11. Home traction can be useful if you have a disc injury or an arthritic condition in your spine that is causing chronic or recurring leg or arm pain. If you have low-back and leg pain, try the traction-with-a-chair technique explained in this chapter.

12. Constipation as a cause of backache can be prevented in many cases by drinking several glasses of water each day, by eating foods that contain roughage, by having regular toilet hours, and by taking regular exercises.

13. The structural integrity of your bones, joints, discs, and ligaments depends upon an adequate intake of all the essential food elements; so make sure that you follow a good all-round diet.

8

Overcoming Backache
at the End of the Day

Just about everyone will have a certain amount of backache at the end of a long day, even when the back and spine are normal. And nothing can spoil an evening out like the dragging fatigue of a nagging backache, the twentieth century's most frustrating ailment. But there is something that you can do *now* to obtain some immediate relief from your symptoms if you have job-related aches and pains.

Basically, there are two types of after-work backache: one type results from lack of exercise and movement during work, and the other type results from excessive use of muscles and joints. The type of backache you have will determine the steps you will need to take to obtain relief.

Actually, prolonged sitting or standing in unchanging postures is probably the most common cause of after-work backache, since the type of work most people do will require such posture. And postural strains in which the joints are not put through a full and varied range of movement are more likely to cause backache than heavy muscular work that allows a great deal of movement. Furthermore, work which requires a certain amount of muscular effort will stimulate the blood circulation to aid in preventing the aching fatigue that results from the accumulation of waste products in the muscles.

Of course, persons who perform an excessive amount of heavy muscular work will very often experience a backache from overwork; and if the individual is unaccustomed to the work, he may develop an acute backache that will compel him to end the day prematurely.

Obviously, the individual who develops backache from heavy muscular exertion will need all the rest he can get before beginning another day. But persons who have a postural-type backache resulting from inadequate movement or exercise will need a little light exercise at the end of the day to relieve the binding fatigue of sagging muscles and joints.

Persons suffering from either type of backache can, of course, benefit from moist heat applications and massage.

Determine the type of backache you have and then follow one of the routines outlined below. They are easy and simple to do, and they should prove to be effective in relieving your backache.

THE BACKACHE OF ALL-DAY SITTING OR STANDING

If you have spent the day working over a desk, sorting mail, painting a building, standing at a blackboard, sitting in school, or turning a screw on an assembly line, then the chances are that you will get more relief from your backache by taking a little exercise than by resting. A swim, a game of handball, a gym workout, or some of the exercises described in Chapters 12 or 13, for example, if taken immediately after work so that you will have a couple of hours to relax before supper, will provide the type of exercise you need to restore your body to a dynamic, functional state. When exercise stimulates the heart rate and respiration, all of the body's physiological processes are stepped up, and the increase in the circulation of blood, along with the chemical changes brought about in preparing the body for physical activity, will literally rejuvenate your sluggish body to make you feel a hundred percent better.

No matter how "fagged out" you feel when you leave the office today, try a little exercise and see if you do not feel a great deal better. I use exercise regularly to snap me out of the lethargy that will sometimes engulf me after a long day of sitting at my desk, and it always seems to restore my strength. I have recommended after-work exercise to a number of business men and office personnel who complained of fatigue and backache at the end of each day, and not one of them has ever said that it did not help. Many, in fact, reported a complete disappearance of a backache they had previously thought they had to "live with."

Case of a Typical Office Worker

One man, a very busy accountant, worked long hours at his desk six days a week in order to keep his books up-to-date. When he closed his office each night, his back ached and his hips were stiff from sitting. And as the months and years of desk work in a sitting position passed into decades, a shortening of the muscles on the front of his hips made it uncomfortable for him to stand erect for very long (which by itself is a cause of backache), and he was developing a gait like that of an astronaut who has just come down from a couple of weeks in orbit in a nose cone. When he got home from the office, supper was always "waiting," so he went directly to the dining room to eat. Now we all know that you do not have to exercise to have a big appetite, and the more we eat the bigger our appetite becomes, since the stomach stretches to accommodate the large volume of food. And, of course, the larger the stomach becomes, the more we have to eat to satisfy our appetite. Thus, when our overweight accountant finally got up from the supper table, he could barely do more than make it to his favorite TV chair where he sat for two or three more hours before going to bed. When morning came, he always had trouble waking up, and as he became more and more sedentary, he became more sluggish. "Doc," he said, "I'm tired all the time. I just can't seem to get enough sleep, and this backache is driving me crazy. Maybe I'm working too hard." How many people do you know who fit this picture? What about yourself?

I advised the accountant to take the rest-break exercises described in Chapter 10 a couple of times a day, and then to take a little light exercise before eating a *smaller* supper. He took several of the exercises described in Chapter 12, including exercise "A" in Group 2, and exercise "A" in Group 3, for development of back and abdominal muscles and to stretch his hamstrings and hip flexors. Six weeks after he began the exercises, he was leaner, more vigorous, and happier.

"I even took my wife dancing last night," he told me one day with a grin.

Many Types of Exercise Available

There are, of course, many good exercises that you can do to wake your body up physically. Jumping rope, for example, when done in the "professional" style of a boxer, can be a fine and challenging exercise that both husband and wife can do. I know several business men who have developed the rope-jumping skill of a boxer, and they are always willing to give a demonstration for skeptical friends. Riding a bicycle is another good way to combine exercise and recreation.

If you ever get into a rut of sedentary living that forces you into that vicious cycle of inactivity, fatigue, and "I-don't-feel-like-exercising" way of life, you may find yourself adding to your fatigue and your backache (and your overweight) by overeating, overresting, and oversleeping. When this happens, you may feel that you are not getting enough rest—not because you actually need more rest, but because your body is as sluggish as a clogged-up fishing reel.

Of course, any exercise you do for stimulating or "loosening up" purposes should be enough to warmup your muscles and to increase your heart rate and respiration. But do not do so much that you become physically exhausted. If you are a beginner at exercise, you should begin very lightly and increase the amount of exercise you do over a period of several weeks. You should enjoy your exercise, and it should not be "hard" or painful.

If you can, follow your exercise with a little massage over the muscles of your back. Anyone can apply the massage if the simplified techniques described in Chapter 7 are used.

Your exercise and massage should then be followed by a hot shower, which should be gradually turned down to a comfortable cold.

The combined effects of the exercise, massage, and shower should make you feel alive, relaxed, and refreshed—and you will be able to eat your supper without the "knots" in your stomach and back that develop from a day of tension and harassment.

If you have trouble getting to sleep each night, you might try soaking in a tub of warm water just before retiring. But you should make sure that your body is not chilled by exposure to cold air or cold sheets when you leave the bath. (See "Relaxing for Sleep" in Chapter 11.)

Persons who take a little regular exercise and who observe the rules of good posture and correct lifting given in Part II of this book will be less likely to have after-work backache. There are, however, many types of employment in which a certain amount of backache cannot be avoided; but if you know what to do, it can be greatly alleviated at the end of the day.

If you decide that your backache is being caused more by "nerves" than by physical strain, you will want to read Chapter 11 on "What to Do About Nervous Backache."

THE BACKACHE OF OVEREXERTION

If you finish a long day loading or unloading trucks, digging ditches, shoveling snow, working in a construction crew, landscaping your lawn, or doing any kind of work in which heavy muscular exertion is called for, you may end up with a backache; and if you are unaccustomed to such work, your backache may be acute.

Since your back muscles have already been overworked by the day's labor, you need rest rather than exercise, so you will probably want to get home as soon as possible to lie down.

Eight Steps to Relieve Backache From Overwork

Here are eight important steps to be taken in relieving backache caused by overwork:

1. Have someone apply moist heat to your back for about 20 minutes. (See "Moist Heat Is Best" in Chapter 7.)
2. Follow the application of heat with stroking massage. "A Simple Technique for Massaging the Back" in Chapter 7

will give you all the instructions you need.

3. Then stand up and bend your trunk forward and from side to side for several repetitions. This will aid the heat and massage in pumping out the irritating waste products that have accumulated in your back muscles.

4. Repeat the application of heat and massage if your backache is acute.

5. Get down on your hands and knees and lift your back up and down in order to loosen up your vertebrae; that is, lift your back up like a camel and then drop it down like a sway-backed horse. See Figures 6 and 7.

6. Follow this routine with a hot shower that is gradually reduced to a cool shower.

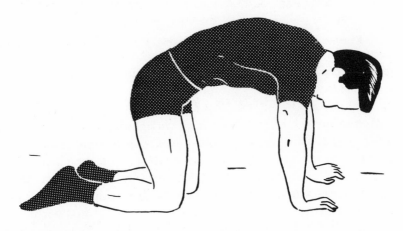

Figure 6:   Relieving a stiff back. Position 1, Exercise 5

7. After your body has been dried with a towel, have someone apply a skin-warming liniment (such as oil of wintergreen) to your back before you get dressed.

8. Make sure that your back muscles are not chilled by exposure to cold air.

Things to Watch in Heavy Exertion

Always try to avoid working too long in heavy work that you are not accustomed to doing. If you take a new job calling for a

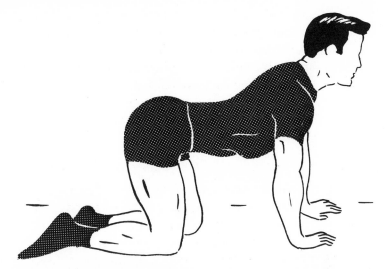

Figure 7:   Relieving a stiff back. Position 2, Exercise 5

great deal of muscular effort, try to start out by working only half a day for the first few days, especially if you are not in good physical condition. One of the worst backaches I have ever had occurred at the age of 16 after I had worked all day at a new job in a bowling alley setting up pins—and I was in good shape physically.

I treated a right-handed patient recently who had developed a severe backache in the muscles on the left side of his lower back after he had spent an entire day bowling, and he had not bowled any at all for 10 sedentary years. Do not be so foolish. Begin lightly in any unaccustomed activity calling for physical exertion, even if it is sport or recreation.

In a great many cases, when the muscles have been overworked in labor or exercise, a little light muscular contraction following such heavy work may aid in preventing an extremely painful muscle reaction. Olympic athletes, for example, who have just finished a running or swimming race will sometimes "taper off" their effort by gradually reducing their activity before they stop altogether. They do this, of course, so that the continued light and slow muscular contractions will pump enough blood through the fatigued muscles to remove most of the irritating waste products that have accumulated from the more rapid and intense contractions. This is why the eight steps outlined for relieving the backache of overexertion include a little light bending exercise.

In any event, if you should overwork to the point of finishing the day with an acute backache, a little light muscular contraction following the application of heat and massage will help to cut down on excessive soreness and stiffness the next day. Otherwise, you just spend the evening resting.

Summary

1. If you finish each day with a backache that has resulted from the type of work in which there is little moving around and only a small amount of muscular activity, your aches and pains will probably vanish with a little all-round exercise right after work. But if you perform heavy labor all day, your backache will respond best to rest, heat, and massage.

2. The 8 simple steps outlined in this chapter will tell you how to relieve backache caused by overwork.

3. When occasions arise that compel you to indulge in heavy, unaccustomed muscular effort that results in acute backache, it is best to follow heat and massage with light, pumping muscular contractions in order to aid the blood circulation in flushing out accumulated waste products.

4. Try to avoid "temporary" jobs that call for heavy, unaccustomed muscular effort. And be careful not to overdo it in strenuous sports or recreation that you do not participate in regularly.

5. When you begin a new job that requires a great deal of exertion or an awkward posture, begin lightly and increase the amount of work you do from day to day until you become accustomed to the job.

6. If you want a simple, entertaining exercise that will increase your heart rate and respiration for a physical awakening, try jumping rope or riding a bicycle.

part II

How to prevent backache at home and on the job

9

How to Build
Healthy Posture

Of all the causes of simple back-
ache that are not related to structural disorders in the spine, mechanical strains caused by bad sitting, standing, or lying-down
postures would probably head the list—and, of course, this would
include the stress and strain of bad working postures. Thus, *it will
be necessary to cultivate good posture and to avoid bad working
postures if backache is to be prevented.*

In a recent survey of 9,000 back patients of two large hospitals,
postural deficiencies were found to be responsible for backache
in 80 percent of the cases! So you can see that the information
contained in this chapter will be of special importance in your
program of backache prevention.

Maintaining good posture is simple enough in itself, but you
will need special instructions in assuming correct posture under
various conditions. A chair that you use regularly, for example,
should meet certain specifications for working or for resting, and

it should be adapted to your height and body build, and so on. Even lying in bed at night can be done more effectively if you know what postures to assume in the various positions.

In addition to instructions in building good posture, there is a set of simple, easy-to-do postural exercises at the end of this chapter that are designed to retrain the muscles of persons who have habitually bad posture.

If you do the exercises in Chapters 12 or 13, you will, of course, experience an automatic improvement in your posture, and the increased strength of your muscles will make it easier for you to stand and sit erect without fatigue. But good, dynamic posture that can be maintained day after day in everything you do must be acquired by constant observation of the rules of sitting and standing correctly. And you must cultivate a "relaxed" posture that will enhance your performance in work or play.

Your Best Posture Is an Individual Matter

Although there are certain general rules to be followed in developing a standard for good posture, no two people have exactly the same posture. It would be foolish to try to force everyone to stand the same way. Differences in bone structure, muscular development, habits, and even eye sight, for example, can result in unusual posture that is normal for the individual, and attempts to change such harmless deviation from the ideal posture could result in many aches and pains as well as fatigue. Persons who back up to a wall and walk away with their head back and their back flat could not possibly hope to maintain such posture longer than five or ten minutes before tiring. And just as soon as something else occupies their mind, their overtensed muscles relax and they have forgotten all about trying to maintain such an exaggerated posture.

Practical Rules for Good Posture

For good posture to be effective, it must be habitual, and it must not require such pronounced muscular contraction that you must concentrate 24 hours a day in order to keep certain muscles tensed and certain muscles relaxed.

Thus, *practical posture must be the result of simple efforts to stand straight in a comfortable and semi-relaxed position in which there is no strain on muscles, joints, or ligaments.* In this way, the posture you assume becomes useful and functional; and after a short time of making a conscious effort to stand correctly, the posture is maintained largely by muscle tone and natural reflexes.

Persons who think that it is easier to slouch than to stand erect are mistaken. There is a great deal more strain on muscles, joints, and ligaments when you stand with your shoulders drooping and your spine bending than there is when you stand with your shoulders back and your spine erect. Once good posture becomes habitual, you will not even be aware of the action of the muscles in your back. But if you develop habitually poor posture, you will be plagued with all kinds of aches and pains, and your muscles will have to work *harder* to keep your unbalanced spine erect!

Of course, there are certain types of work in which it is impossible to maintain good, balanced posture, and I have the greatest sympathy for workers who must maintain bent postures day in and day out. A housewife, for example, who does a great deal of ironing for a large family may suffer from postural backache. I ironed a couple of pairs of shorts myself in an emergency, and the backache I developed in my neck and between my shoulder blades doubled my respect for the overworked housewife who has children to look after.

Bad Posture Is Unhealthy, Ugly and Self-Deprecating!

If you remember the lesson in anatomy you received in Part I of this book, you know that there are certain front to back curves in your spine that are provided by nature to balance your bodyweight and to permit movement in your trunk. Only persons who are totally ignorant of spinal anatomy would attempt to completely flatten out normal spinal curves by lying on a floor or by standing against a wall. See examples of good and bad posture in Figure 8.

When poor posture occurs, the normal curves of the spine become greatly exaggerated. Even persons who do not know what a normal spine should look like can see that bad posture is ugly

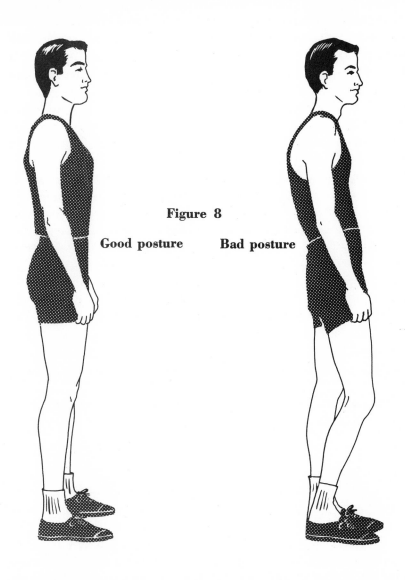

Figure 8

Good posture   **Bad posture**

and unhealthy in appearance. The part of the spine between the shoulders, for example, may be so rounded that the individual looks hump-backed. And the head may project so far out over a flattened chest that it looks as if the rib cage has caved in. In the

lower part of the back, the lumbar spine and hips bend forward
to flatten out the buttocks and cause a "pot belly" below the
beltline. The entire body is so out of balance that there is a constant struggle between gravity and the muscles to keep the body
from folding up like a paper skeleton—and the results are never
healthy.

Thus, aside from aches and pains, sagging posture has a devas-
tating effect on the appearance of the body.

GOOD POSTURE WITHOUT STRONG MUSCLES?

There is, of course, more to good posture than just keeping the
spine properly balanced. You must also keep your muscles adequately developed. We have all seen people whose abdomens
sagged grotesquely and whose back muscles ached constantly
because of inadequate exercise, even though they stood "straight."
Thus, *well-developed abdominal muscles are just as important
as strong back muscles.* And muscular support for an elevated rib
cage adds as much to the appearance of good posture as a properly aligned spine. So you can see that it will be important for
you to continue doing the exercises described in this book, even
when your posture is "good."

THE CONSEQUENCES OF BAD POSTURE

When the body begins to sag because of poor posture and weak
muscles, a great many unhealthy things begin to happen. The
normal curves of the spine, as you just learned, become greatly
exaggerated, resulting in a round-shouldered and sway-backed
standing position that places considerable strain on the joints of
the spine. Normally, the bodyweight is supported by the intervertebral discs when the spine is erect and balanced, and the
knocks and bangs of walking and running are absorbed by these
cushion-like shock absorbers. But when the normal curves of
the spine are thrown out of balance, much of the stress and strain
of weight bearing is shifted to muscles, joints, and ligaments,
causing a backache that might be accompanied by arthritis, nerve
pains, muscle spasm, disc degeneration, and other disorders resulting from abused spinal joints. In addition, a forward bending
of the spine shoves the ribs together and down, thus diminishing
the capacity of the thoracic cavity. As a result, the heart and

lungs are squeezed into a smaller working area, and the diaphragm is forced to move farther down in respiration, causing considerable respiratory "embarrassment." Persons who suffer from such poor posture are very often "breathless" after a meal, and they find it difficult to take a deep breath.

When very bad posture is combined with obesity and muscle weakness, there may be some danger of abnormal pressures interfering with the normal function of the abdominal and pelvic organs. In some cases, for example, organs may become heavy and congested with blood as a result of interference with venous blood flow, or they may become ischemic (bloodless) because of interference with arterial blood flow. In any event, every possible measure should be taken to prevent the development of a bulging, sagging abdomen that results from overeating and inadequate exercise.

There is some medical literature being published that contends that posture by itself has nothing to do with organic health. This might be true as far as the average person is concerned, since most of us display only mild structural distortions in bad posture. But there seems to be no doubt among medical authorities that very bad posture in combination with obesity and muscle weakness can affect the internal organs adversely, especially when the abdomen hangs down in front like a bag of melons. In any event, *all medical authorities agree that bad posture is a common cause of backache!* And when posture is bad, there is a greater likelihood of "slipped discs," bone defects, and other structural disorders causing trouble.

When you total up the joint disorders, the nerve pains, the circulatory disturbances, the weaknesses, and the ligamentous and muscular aches and pains that can and do occur from prolonged postural distortions, however minor they may appear to be, it is inconceivable that any intelligent, thinking adult would allow his physical condition to "go to pot," so to speak. Yet, there are millions of people who rarely, if ever, get down on the floor and do simple situps.

Bad Posture a Cause of Constant Backache

I see people every day who stand and sit in such bad postures that they suffer from backache constantly. I knew a 28-year-old overweight student, for example, who sagged and slumped so bad that no part of his back was free from aches and pains. His neck ached from the constant tension on muscles that held his sagging head up. The joints in his back between his shoulder blades ached from being stretched apart as his spine gradually collapsed into a hump. And the muscles supporting his shoulder girdle ached because of increasing roundness of his shoulders. In the lower part of his back, his sway-backed spine ached because of a jamming together of the vertebral joints, and his lumbar muscles ached because of the constant tension placed on them by the off-center weight of his pot belly in front. Even his hips ached because of a tilting of his pelvis. And his aches and pains were growing steadily worse! Physically, he looked and felt like an old man. He was literally one big walking ache. It was not until he began to experience a little sharp pain that would "shoot" down an arm or a leg occasionally that he became alarmed enough to do something about his posture. I recommended the postural exercises at the end of this chapter, and many of the exercises in Chapter 12. After three months, he was many pounds lighter, his spine was straighter, and he was nearly free of aches and pains. Best of all, he looked 20 years younger.

Reasons of personal appearance alone are enough to warrant the use of a regular program of posture-improving exercises, but *freedom from the slavery of backache should present a final and conclusive argument in favor of good posture and a little regular exercise for preventive purposes.*

How to Assume Good Standing and Walking Posture

Although we cannot all stand exactly alike, we can all observe the same basic rules in maintaining posture that will place our joints in natural, balanced positions.

The first thing you should do, of course, is to make a simple effort to stand "tall," as though you were trying to increase your height a little. You should then lift your chest very slightly so that there will be just enough tension on your muscles to hold your rib cage up. Move your shoulders back just a little in order to keep your shoulder girdle from sagging. Pull your stomach in a little so that your abdominal wall will be flat. (Try tightening up your belt a notch, and then hold your stomach in to keep the belt from being too tight.) *The ability to flatten out your abdomen by lifting up your abdominal muscles is an important key to good posture and good body mechanics.* If you have a tendency to be sway-backed, you can tuck your hips under a little to prevent the development of an exaggerated lumbar curve.

Stand and walk with your toes pointed fairly straight ahead and lift your arches up a little so that your weight is supported on the front, back, and outside portions of your feet. In other words, *do not let your ankles roll in to flatten your arches against the floor.* You already know, from reading Part I of this book, that relaxed arches in a slue-footed stance can cause bad posture, which can cause backache.

Occasionally assume a correct standing position as an exercise and then rock back on your heels slightly so that the change in your center of balance will tighten up your thigh muscles. Let your arms hang loosely at your sides and keep your head and neck in a comfortable position with your chin drawn back a little.

You may exaggerate the positions of good posture for exercise purposes, but the muscular tension needed to maintain good posture must be just enough to permit its use habitually. If you over-tense your muscles you will soon tire, and a great deal of concentration will be needed to maintain your posture.

Good posture should be dynamic; that is, you should be able to move about freely and efficiently and still maintain correct posture. Static posture in which muscle tension holds the joints in the same position all day, or in which there is little or no movement, can, by itself, cause backache. If you have a job that requires a lot of standing or sitting, try to break postural tension occasionally by moving about, by bending your trunk, or even by lying down if you can.

How to Have a Healthy Posture Lying Down

Since we spend a large part of our life lying down, it is important that we carry our good posture to bed with us.

The first thing you should do, of course, is to make sure that you have the right kind of mattress; that is, it should be firm enough to keep your spine from sagging, but not so hard that it cannot mold itself to the normal curves of the spine. (See "A Firm Mattress Is Important" in Chapter 7.)

Avoid Sleeping On Your Stomach

Try to avoid sleeping on your stomach, since most beds will give enough to let your lower back sag a little. It would, in fact, be a good idea to try to cultivate the habit of sleeping on your back or your side (even if sleeping face down does not cause you any discomfort at the present time) so that you will not have trouble with your sleeping posture when you do begin to have a little back trouble. If you prefer to sleep face down, do not use a pillow under your head; and if your lower back is uncomfortable in this position, bend one knee up and out on the side toward which your face is turned. A thin pillow placed under the edge of your abdomen on the front side will keep your spine from sagging. If you have back trouble and you must lie face down for the application of heat and massage, or if you "cannot sleep any other way," you might be able to rest all right with a pillow under your pelvis. But remember that the most comfortable way to rest in bed when you have suffered a low-back injury is to lie flat on your back with a pillow under both knees.

How to Sleep on Your Side

If you sleep on your side, use a thick pillow under your head and bend both knees. If you do not have back trouble, your top knee may rest on top of your bottom knee. But if you do have back trouble, place a pillow between your knees so that both thighs will rest parallel to each other. Persons who have large hips and a small waist may have to place a thin pillow under their side in order to keep their spine from sagging when lying in a side position.

The Best Sleeping Position

The best way to sleep, of course, as far as keeping the spine properly aligned, is on your back. In this position, you should use only a thin pillow—or no pillow at all—under your head so that your neck will be in line with the rest of your spine. Persons who are hump-backed or who have thick shoulders, however, may have to use a fairly thick pillow under their head when lying on their back in order to keep their head from tilting backward.

If your lower back is uncomfortable when you lie flat on your back, a thin pillow placed under both knees will help. (When you lie on your back with your legs flat on the mattress, certain muscles hooking up between the thigh bones and the lumbar spine may cause your lower back to arch up a little, especially if you have prominent buttocks. You may not notice this unless you have back trouble, in which case a pillow placed under both knees will relieve the strain.)

Do not sit up in bed with your legs straight out in front and flat on the mattress; and do not lie on your back with your heels supported in such a way that there is no support under the back of your legs. A sagging mattress or a hammock will sometimes suspend the legs in this manner.

Persons who sleep on their back with their hands folded over their abdomen sometimes experience a temporary numbness on the little-finger side of their hand and forearm from the pressure of the bed against the ulnar nerve in the elbow. Changing the position of the arms, or placing a soft pillow under each elbow, will relieve such symptoms.

Good posture in bed requires restful positions in which the joints of the body, especially the spine, are relaxed and aligned without any strain on the ligaments and without any jamming of the joints. If you get up in the mornings with backache, then the chances are that you have bad sleeping posture.

How to Sit Correctly for Your Back's Sake

Since most of us sit more than we stand each day, we are just as likely to develop bad posture or to get a backache from incorrect sitting as we are from incorrect standing. So the rules of good posture should not be disregarded when we sit down.

If you spend a lot of time typing or working at a desk in a tense, erect posture, you should use a simple straight-backed chair that is not too heavily padded. Sit far enough back in the chair that your buttocks touch the back portion of the chair, and then sit erect with a slight arch in your lower back and your

weight distributed evenly on both buttocks. You can check your
sitting posture occasionally by leaning backward against the
chair back. Of course, you will have to tilt your head down or to
one side to do your work, but if you will take frequent breaks and
reverse the working posture of your neck you may be able to
avoid excessive fatigue or tension. (See Figure 9 for correct sitting posture.)

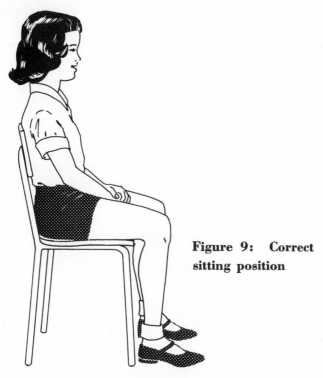

**Figure 9:   Correct
sitting position**

Persons who do a lot of handwriting or drawing should have
a fairly high desk that has a slanted top so that there will be less
slumping from bracing the elbows on the desk—and the chair
should be pulled up close to the desk.

A chair with an adjustable back in which an upper and lower
portion can be moved up or down to fit the back of the individual
would be helpful to office workers and students who may sit in
semi-relaxed positions. The upper portion of the chair back should
be hollowed out to fit the upper back, while the lower portion
should be rounded out to fit into the lower back.

Remember that the mind can absorb more than the seat can endure, so correct sitting posture can be especially important for students.

How to Select the Right Kind of Chair

If you do a great deal of reading, or if you must sit for a long time sewing, convalescing, or doing some kind of work in which you are not using a desk and in which you may sit relaxed, your chair should have arm rests, and the chair-back should be slanted backward 15 or 20 degrees in order to relieve tension on the muscles of the spine.

When possible, *the height of each chair should be adjusted for the individual so that both feet rest flat on the floor while the thighs and legs are at right angles to each other.* If the chair is too high and the feet dangle, the pressure of the edge of the chair behind the knees might damage the sciatic nerve and cause numbness in both legs, and sitting will be very uncomfortable. If the chair seat is too low, the knees will be thrust upward (when both feet are flat on the floor), which may cause the spine to slump and the lower back to reverse its normal curve.

A chair seat may be hollowed out a little so that it can mold itself to the shape of the thighs and buttocks for additional comfort. If the back of the chair slants backward, the front portion of the chair seat may be slanted upward a little to prevent the buttocks from slipping forward.

Chairs with tilting backs, such as those used in airliners, barber shops, and buses, would probably provide better support if the entire chair could be tilted backward as a unit; that is, if the seat, the chair-back, and the foot-rest could be tilted backward at adjusted, fixed angles, thus maintaining the same support recommended for sitting in an upright position.

Arm rests on chairs should be just high enough to support the arms without a push or pull on the shoulder joints.

Too much sitting day after day can result in a shortening of certain muscles that attach between the thigh and the lower spine in front, and between the thigh and leg in back, which can cause backache when these muscles are stretched on prolonged standing. This type of backache can be prevented, however, by occasionally lying across your bed with your legs locked out and your feet resting on the floor in order to stretch your hip flexors, and by lying on the floor and raising one leg at a time (as far as you can with your leg straight) in order to stretch your hamstrings. (See the exercises in Group 3 of Chapter 12.)

How to Avoid "Motorist's Spine"

If the back portion of your automobile or truck seat is not molded to fit the normal curves of your spine, you can very easily add a little temporary support for long trips. The back of the average automobile seat, for example, is usually slanted so far backward that the entire spine rounds itself into a "C" shape when you reach forward to grasp the steering wheel with both hands. And this can cause a lumbosacral strain that is known as "motorist's spine."

The first thing you should do in fitting your car seat to your back is to suspend a small cushion (by cords) from the top of the seat-back so that it will hang in just the right position to fit into the hollow of your lower back. In most cases, the cushion will hang about 6 inches from the bottom of the seat. If you feel as though you need additional support for the upper portion of your spine, you can suspend a second cushion that will hang near the top of the seat-back. The second cushion, of course, should be wide and flat so that it will support the entire width of the shoulders.

You may have to experiment a little to find the right level and the correct size and shape for your suspended car-seat cushions, but if you are constantly traveling it should be worth the effort. Some drivers may prefer to simply fold up a towel that can be placed behind the lower back. In any event, if you know how the normal curves of the spine are constructed (and you should if you read Chapter 3 of this book), you will have no trouble adding a little additional support for your back when necessary.

The next thing you should do to prevent "motorist's spine" is to move your car seat forward so that you will be sitting close enough to the gas pedal to place your foot on it with your knee bent. When you have to straighten out your leg in reaching for the gas pedal, the tightened tendons on the back of your leg transmit a torsion strain to your right sacroiliac joint, which can result in a chronic sacroiliac strain. If you combine inadequate back support with straight-leg operation of the gas pedal on long trips, you may experience an acute backache at the end of each day of travel.

The driver's seat in most buses and trucks is constructed so that the driver can sit erect with his lower leg nearly straight up and down while his foot is on the gas pedal, and the seat is nearly always firm. The same seating arrangement should also be placed in automobiles, but most American motorists demand the highly cushioned, long, and sleek type of seats that are designed more for looks than for comfort.

When a car seat is too soft or too hard, pressure against the back of the thigh in bad sitting postures can damage the sciatic nerve, resulting in "driver's thigh," or an inability to lift the toes on the affected side when walking. Try to sit so that there is not an excessive amount of pressure against the back of your thighs.

A knee rest on the outside of the right knee will relieve the hip and knee strain caused by a tendency for the leg to swing to the right while the foot is on the accelerator.

Cross-Leg and "Saturday Night Paralysis"

Students who sit for long periods of time with their legs crossed will very often suffer from a painless form of "foot drop" that disappears when the crossed-leg sitting is discontinued. I experienced this condition myself while I was attending college; and until I found out what was wrong, I felt sure that I was coming down with some terrible disease of the nervous system. (The portion of the sciatic nerve passing down behind the knee is not adequately protected by overlying muscles, so that the pressure of the supporting knee literally presses the nerve against the bone of the crossed-over thigh.)

Persons who sit too long with one or both of their arms draped over the back of a hard chair or bench sometimes suffer pressure-damage in the nerves of the arm. The resulting paralysis, most often seen in persons who sleep off a drunk on a park bench, has been appropriately labeled "Saturday night paralysis" in medical text books.

Teenagers sometimes develop the very bad habit of draping one leg over the arm of a chair, and one arm over the back of the chair. Obviously, such sitting posture, if maintained for hours at a time, could damage the nerves in both the arm and the leg as well as put a curvature-causing strain on the spine.

How To Alleviate "Tractor Back" Backache

Workers who ride around on tractors all day may experience a backache that is different from that suffered by a "worn-out" motorist. A farmer or a heavy-equipment operator, for example, might be bounced and jarred by the movement of his machine over rough ground, and if he is not sitting on a cushioned surface, his spine will be forced to absorb much of the shock transmitted through the seat.

Obviously, the first thing you should do if you ride a tractor is to sit on a cushion. Then, if you have back trouble, it might help to wear a wide belt similar to those worn by motorcycle drivers. Of course, all of the rules of proper sitting should also be observed. If the spine is allowed to slump during a bumpy ride, the danger of strain from bad posture would be greatly increased, and the tailbone might be subjected to painful injury.

If you spend long hours operating machinery which compels you to work under the stress and strain of working levers while keeping constantly alert, much of the fatigue, tension, and backache you experience will be unavoidable, since they may be "occupational hazards." You can, however, reduce your discomfort by observing the rules of good posture, by taking a little regular exercise, and by utilizing the end-of-the-day treatment routines offered in Chapter 8.

Workers who have spinal arthritis or a "slipped disc" may find it impossible to endure the constant jarring of riding heavy equipment.

Four Beneficial Posture Drills

Since good posture depends to a large extent upon muscle control, get the whole family together occasionally and go through the following drills.

(Drill 1) Lifting the Chest

Lift your chest as high as you can with a deep breath. Keep your back straight and pull in your abdomen as you inhale. Do not do this exercise more than two or three times, lest you become dizzy from upsetting the oxygen-carbon dioxide balance in your blood. When you are breathless from having performed a little exercise, however, you can practice this drill more extensively.

(Drill 2) Pulling In the Abdomen

Pull your abdomen in as though you were trying to squeeze your stomach. In order to make sure that you use your stomach muscles rather than your chest muscles, try exhaling during this exercise.

Next, exhale and hold your breath so that you can draw your stomach in by lifting your diaphragm. This will take a little practice. Just try to suck your stomach up into your chest.

(Drill 3) Squaring the Shoulders

Lift your chest up and throw your shoulders back as though you were trying to squeeze your shoulder blades together; then lift your shoulders up toward your ears in a shrugging movement. Let your arms hang perfectly relaxed throughout both parts of this exercise.

(Drill 4) Loosening the Spine

Get down on your hands and knees for this three-position exercise. In *position 1*, arch your back down as far as you can (like a sway-backed horse) by contracting your back muscles. Go from there to *position 2*, in which you lift your spine up to what you feel is a neutral or straight position. Then go to *position 3* by arching your back up as high as you can (like a hump-backed camel), with vigorous contraction of your abdominal muscles. (If you have a small child, try letting him ride your back occasionally for added resistance.)

These four drills, simple as they are, will develop the muscle control you need to keep a little tension on key muscles in maintaining good posture. Do several repetitions in each exercise three or four times a week, or as often as you like.

Exercise Pays Off in Maintaining Good Posture

The older we become, the more important it is to take a little regular exercise in maintaining good posture. Muscles that are

too weak to hold the body erect without becoming fatigued will
eventually give under the *pull of gravity*, especially when the
intervertebral discs begin to deteriorate with age. When the spinal
joints are supported by the tone of well-developed muscles on all
sides, however, good posture is much easier. And putting the
joints through a full range of extension and flexion (as in Drill
4) will maintain flexibility.

Do not fool yourself into thinking that you always get adequate exercise on the job just because the work you do leaves
you tired and aching at the end of the day. Actually, there is no
beneficial exercise at all in office-type activity or in assembly-line
factory work, and the muscles, rather than getting stronger for
the performance of such work, become weaker. A typist, for
example, who finishes each day with aching shoulders and a sore
neck, may experience greater fatigue and pain as the days pass
if the muscles are not exercised in order to strengthen them for
the simple task of supporting the trunk and the shoulders in
static postures.

So even if your posture does appear to be "good" when you
stand before a mirror, you should take a little regular exercise
if you want to keep it that way. But remember that there is more
to good posture than just having strong muscles. You will have
to walk, stand, sit, and sleep correctly if you want to avoid postural backache.

Summary

1. Although well-developed muscles are important in maintaining good posture, certain basic rules of sitting and
   standing must be observed constantly if good posture is
   to be habitual and effective and prevent postural backache.
2. It is much easier to maintain good posture than it is to
   endure bad posture. Furthermore, persons who have well-
   balanced posture have less backache and fewer aches and
   pains.
3. Basically, good posture consists of standing *tall* with just
   enough tension on the muscles to hold the shoulders and
   chest up and to keep the abdomen flat. Try to stand and
   walk with your toes pointed fairly straight ahead, and

lift your arches up enough to keep your ankles from rolling in.

4. Always try to keep the normal curves of your spine properly aligned when you are sitting, standing, or lying down.

5. Generally speaking, lying face-down is the worst way to rest in bed, while lying on your back with your knees slightly bent (supported by a thin pillow) is the best way to rest as far as the spine is concerned.

6. When you sit, either sit erect and voluntarily maintain the normal curves of your spine, or use a chair which molds itself to the curves of your back when you lean backward in relaxation.

7. Always avoid using a chair that is so high that the edge of the seat cuts into the back of your thighs. Try to keep both feet flat on the floor with your thighs and legs at right angles to each other.

8. Make sure that your automobile seat molds itself to the normal curves of your spine if you travel a great deal. A small cushion or a folded-up towel placed in the hollow of your lower back would be helpful.

9. Get the family together occasionally and go through the posture drills at the end of this chapter.

10

How to Lift Correctly and Avoid Painful Strains

According to the U.S. Public Health Service, about 9 million employed persons each year suffer on-the-job work injuries that are bad enough to require medical attention or to cause restriction in work ability for a day or more. Of the total number of workers injured, the second and third most common causes of injury are falls and one-time lifting or exertion.[1] *And medical records indicate that falls and lifting accidents are the two major causes of back injury!* Thus, good working conditions and observation of basic safety rules, as well as correct techniques in lifting, are just as important in preventing back injury as having strong muscles and a straight spine.

No matter how strong your muscles are, or how good your posture is, you will have to learn to lift correctly if you want to avoid straining your back.

---

[1] *Health Statistics,* U.S. Dept. of Health, Education, and Welfare, Washington, D.C., February, 1963.

Hardly a day goes by that most of us are not required to do a little lifting of some sort. And as you will learn in this chapter, you can hurt your back just as easily by lifting light objects incorrectly as you can by lifting heavy objects! So correct lifting techniques are important, regardless of your physical condition.

If you strengthen your back and legs by doing the barbell squatting and lifting exercises described in Chapter 13, you will automatically acquire much of the strength and skill needed to lift heavy objects correctly. But there are special techniques to be learned in pushing and pulling, as well as in lifting and carrying heavy objects from one place to another, if you are to provide maximum protection for your all-important back and spine.

In addition to lifting correctly and avoiding accidents at home and on the job, workers who have certain types of back trouble can cut down on backache and back injuries by altering working conditions to fit their particular needs. Thus, fitting each worker to his job can be an important part of backache prevention.

This chapter also contains a description of simple rest-break exercises that will reduce on-the-job backache for any kind of worker, thus paying big dividends by increasing production and decreasing disability.

Techniques of Correct Lifting

Practically everyone is aware of the fact that heavy lifting should be done with the legs and not with the back. This is accomplished by keeping the back flat and squatting down for a two-hand grip on the object to be lifted so that the weight may be lifted by straightening the legs in coming to an erect position. (See Exercise 7 in Chapter 13.) When the object is very heavy, you should let it rest down at arm's length in front (right next to your body) after you stand erect with it. (See Figure 10.)

Bodyweight Balance

When you are lifting any object that is heavy enough to require the use of both hands, you should *make sure that your bodyweight is balanced on both feet and that your feet are parallel and comfortably spaced.* If you try to lift a heavy object from the floor with one foot in back of another, or with more weight on

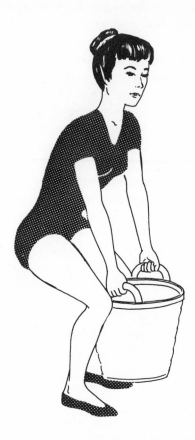

Figure 10:   Keeping the back flat and lifting with the legs

one arm or leg than the other, you could subject your spine to a twist through uneven contraction of the muscles, which might strain a joint or pull a muscle.

Dangers of Lifting With One Hand

It is never a good idea to lift a heavy weight from the floor with one arm, especially when you must strain or bend to the side in making the actual lift. If you do attempt to lift a heavy object (such as a tool box) from the floor with one hand, brace your free hand against your knee on the same side for support in beginning the lift, and then keep your back flat and lift with your legs. When possible, lift the object from a position between your feet and then shift it to one side if you cannot hold it in front with both hands.

Regardless of how small or light an object is, you should always try to lift it correctly; that is, by bending your knees and squatting low with your back flat so that you can lift with your legs. Always face the object you are lifting, and lift in front so that you can center your effort in line with your center of balance. Many people, strong men included, have strained their back by lifting light objects in such awkward and unbalanced positions that the spinal joints are twisted from lack of muscular support or by uneven muscular contraction. This is exactly what happens when a husky worker strains his back by "picking up a pencil."

Both Feet on the Floor

Always stop and plant both feet on the floor before picking up anything! You can hurt your back easily by trying to pick up something as you walk by it, thus straining your spine by twisting or leaning to one side as you go by the object you are reaching for. You cannot afford to be in such a hurry.

Never stand on one leg and bend forward, especially when you are leaning over to pick up an object.

When both feet are planted on the floor and your muscles are "set" in correct lifting techniques, you are less likely to strain your back in lifting heavy objects than you are in lifting light objects incorrectly.

Majority Cause of Back Strains

By far, the majority of acute back strains occur as a result of bending over and lifting with a rounded back. A paint salesman, for example, leaned over to pick up a case of paint and fell to the floor when a sharp pain struck him across his lower back. It took him three weeks to recover. "Next time," he said, "I'll lower my behind instead of my head."

After you have picked up an object, you should lower it with the same correct technique that you used in lifting it. You can strain your back just as easily when you put an object down as you can when you pick it up.

You should never lift or lower an object with your legs straight (unless you are taking a carefully controlled exercise). It is even more dangerous to attempt to lift or lower an object while you are standing on one leg.

Always plan beforehand how you will lift an object and then what you will do with it. Do not be like the "lame brain" who strained his back severely while trying to decide whether he should place a 100-pound motor on a rickety stool or a patched-up chair after he had already lifted the motor. If you are wise, you will not be lifting such heavy and awkward-to-handle objects as a motor without help—and then only if you are compelled to do so.

Do not try to lift an object from the floor to a table by swinging it from side to side for momentum. First lift the object correctly by standing erect with the object down at arm's length in front; then walk up to the table, lift the object up close to your body, and place it on the table. If you want to transfer the object from a lower table to a higher table, and the weight of the object is too heavy for you to lift up with your arms, just squat down in front of the object with your back flat and clamp it to your chest with both arms so that when you stand erect it will be raised to a higher level for the higher table. If you do use this technique of placing a heavy box on top of a high table, try to select a go-between table that is about waist high.

Be careful not to sneeze while lifting or supporting a heavy objects

You might lose control of the lift or suffer a severe strain from the spasmodic action of muscles that are already under tension. As you learned earlier, you can "slip a disc" in simple, uncontrolled sneezing, and this danger is increased if you should sneeze while the discs are being compressed in the act of supporting additional weight. You should also avoid sneezing while in an awkward position or while bending over, especially if you are lifting, pushing, or pulling.

Except in the case of a professional weightlifter, heavy objects should never be jerked from the floor in an attempt to get them to a higher level by using momentum. Painful tears can occur in the muscles and tendons of the back when relaxed muscles are suddenly contracted with a jerk.

If you do lift a fairly heavy object with a technique that calls for speed and momentum, make sure that the object does not strike anything on the way up. More than one worker has injured himself in routine stacking of crates and boxes when a lift was interrupted by striking a shelf or some other obstruction. Workmen who shovel clay sometimes suffer a similar injury ("clay-shoveler's fracture," or a fracture of a portion of a vertebra in the neck or between the shoulders) when the clay sticks to the shovel in attempts to throw the clay to one side or over the shoulder.

Trying to jerk a weight up from the floor with relaxed muscles is dangerous enough, but if the momentum of a rapid lifting movement is interrupted suddenly by an obstruction, by a change in the resistance of the lift, or by an error in timing, a sudden jerk on the muscles can cause a serious back injury.

Do all of your lifting deliberately, carefully, properly, and without speed, and make sure that nothing is in your way. Before lifting any heavy object, first test the weight of the object and then tense your muscles gradually in beginning the lift. Keep an even tension on your muscles during a lift. If you cannot lift an object without jerking it up, it is too heavy for you to lift safely.

The Right Way to Carry a Heavy Object

When possible, you should avoid walking while supporting a heavy object. The seesaw effect on your lower back (as your bodyweight and the weight of the object you are carrying is shifted from one leg to the other) could cause acute back pain if there are joint defects in your lower spine.

If you have to carry a heavy tool box or a large suit case across a room, grip the handle with both hands in front of you and let the box or case rest against the front of your body while carrying it.

When you are carrying an object that is not so heavy that you cannot lift it up into your arms, you may lift it up to the level of your abdomen or higher, but you should always let it rest against your body. *It is very easy to strain your back by trying to hold*

an object away from your body while you are carrying it. A pic-
nicker who carries a dripping ice chest out in front is a good
candidate for back strain—and so is a dressed-up housewife who
is taking out the garbage or carrying around a baby that has wet
diapers.

*Always wear protection when you are handling fairly heavy
objects if you are worried about soiling your clothes.* One of the
most common causes of back strain can be traced to improper
lifting and carrying techniques in which leverage is placed on the
lower back from leverage on the arms out in front, as in trying
to raise a stuck window while leaning over a table or a radiator,
or in trying to carry a heavy object out in front without it touching the body.

For example, a husky warehouse worker came in for treatment
for what was apparently a low-back strain. But when I questioned
him about his activities, he could not recall doing anything that
might have hurt his back—although he added that he had worked
a little Sunday afternoon to help fill an important order. "I don't
see how I could have hurt my back that way, though," he said.
"I do that kind of work every day." With further questioning,
however, I learned that he had on his "Sunday best" trousers
during the work, and he had not worn an apron to protect his
clothing. As a result, he did not let the cartons rest against his
body as he usually did when loading a truck. When X-ray examination revealed a structural defect in his lower spine, it became obvious that the leverage placed on his back in his attempt
to protect his trousers had strained a potentially weak spine.

Moral: You do not have to be a sissy to wear an apron. And do
not get careless in using your back, even if you have never had
back trouble before!

How to Push With Power

When you want to push the family car, move a heavy sofa, or
slide a refrigerator a few feet to sweep up accumulated dust, you
should use a technique of pushing that will permit you to put
your bodyweight into your effort, and you should do it in such
a way that there is no leverage on your lower back.

In pushing a car, for example, you should place both hands on
the back of the car and then step back so that when you lean

down toward the car with your elbows bent your legs and your spine will be aligned for pushing with your legs. The force of the push should be transmitted through your arms with your hands at about shoulder level. If you place your hands too low or too high, a great deal of leverage would be transmitted to your spine, and there would be a greater tendency for you to bend your back in pushing with your arms.

Thus, strong and effective pushing should be done by keeping the back straight and in line with the driving force of the legs, and the body should be tilted toward the object being pushed so that the legs do all the pushing. You never know when you might have to push your car off a busy freeway, so you may need the extra power provided by a correct pushing technique—not to mention protection for your back and spine. (See Figure 11.)

When an object you want to move is too low to push from the shoulder, you may have to pull instead of push. A housewife, for

Figure 11:   Keeping the spine in line with the pushing force of the legs

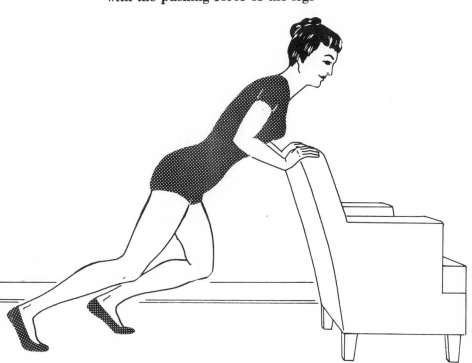

example, who tries to push a mattress across a bed in order to line it up with the springs might be in for trouble. In one instance, a woman leaned over, placed her palms against the edge of the mattress, and tried to move the mattress by shoving with her arms. The only thing that moved was her back, and the lumbosacral strain she suffered made it impossible for her to do any housework for two weeks. I instructed her to *pull* the mattress the next time, but to be cautious and use the correct technique.

You should never try to push a low, heavy piece of furniture by putting your arms down in front of your body in an underhand manner, as though you were trying to raise the hood of your car or throw out the family cat. This would place a tremendous amount of leverage on your shoulders and lower back. Do not use your back as a lever!

How to Pull Without Straining

When you want to pull a heavy object, such as a roped log or a boat trailer, you should assume a position similar to that assumed by athletes in a rope tug-of-war; that is, you should lean away from the object you are pulling so that your arms and trunk will be in line with the force being applied by your legs. Do not let your spine bend forward during heavy pulling, and do most of the pulling by pushing with your legs. As in incorrect pushing techniques, incorrect pulling techniques place too much leverage on the lower back, thus subjecting the lower spine to terrific strain.

You may also exert a pulling force while facing away from the object you are pulling, but this is usually less convenient than facing the object. When you face away from the load, for example, it may be necessary to rig up a harness so that the force can be expressed from the shoulders rather than from the arms. But in either case, the basic technique is about the same; that is, you should pull with the driving force of your legs in line with a straight spine.

Take an Exercise Break Instead of a Coffee Break!

Many factories and offices have found that a "coffee break" in the middle of the afternoon will increase the productivity of employees and cut down on the fatigue that leads to backache. There are many reasons for this, the most important one being that a change from tiring work postures relieves tension on the muscles and joints long enough for recovery from fatigue to take place. And, of course, the stimulating effects of a cup of coffee or a cola drink may give the worker an energetic boost.

There is reason to believe, however, that an "exercise break" might be more effective than a coffee break for factory workers and white-collar office workers who want to prevent the backache of prolonged sitting and standing. And the physiological stimulation of a little "rest-break exercise" might be more effective than a cup of coffee in boosting energy and reducing fatigue.

I read a research abstract taken from a Russian physical-training journal, for example, that said that "rest exercises" taken one and one-half hours after lunch cut down on the number of mistakes made by workers and helped to overcome boredom and to improve emotional health.[2]

It seems logical to assume that a few minutes of exercise in the middle of the afternoon would decrease fatigue and reduce aches and pains by stimulating the circulation of blood. Furthermore, light bending exercises that are designed to put the joints through a full and varied range of movement would relax muscles and relieve jamming and binding of joints that are being forced to work within a limited range of movement. And once the body's physiological processes have been stimulated by exercise, the mind works better, the eye is sharper, and the hand is more efficient.

Anyone who has ever taken a little mild exercise after a tiring day of sitting and standing knows that both mind and body are refreshed by the rejuvenating effects of an increased blood circulation, and the loosening of muscles and joints gets rid of fatiguing stiffness. As far as the back and spine are concerned, nothing is more likely to cause work-distracting backache than unrelieved work routines in which there is little or no movement or change. A janitor, for example, is less likely to have job-related backache than a post office employee who sorts mail all day.

---

[2] *Research Quarterly*, American Association for Health, Physical Education, and Recreation, Washington, D.C., October, 1964.

Thus, employers and employees who want to increase work efficiency and reduce backache should try to organize an afternoon "exercise break." But the exercises should be light and simple, and they should be designed to move the joints through a full range of movement. Of course, participation in such a program would have to be voluntary, but most persons who experience the stimulation of a little mid-afternoon exercise will want to continue such exercise.

Five Simple Rest-Break Exercises

Here are a few simple rest-break exercises that anyone can do:

1. Stand on one leg, while holding on to something for balance, and flex the opposite hip and knee through a full range of movement; that is, bend your knee and lift your thigh up in front as high as you can, and then straighten out your leg until your foot is a few inches above the floor. Contract the muscles on the front of your thigh as you lock your leg down in front. Do not let your foot touch the floor during the exercise, and do several repetitions with each leg.

   This "leg-pumping exercise" will pump the blood through the big thigh muscles, and it will loosen up your hip joints.

2. Next do trunk-bending exercises in which you bend forward and from side to side with your hands on your hips. Do not bend too far; stay within a comfortable range of movement.

3. If possible, include this vertebrae-loosening, disc-expanding exercise: Get down on your hands and knees like a four-legged animal and arch your back down like a sway-backed horse and then up like a hump-backed camel. Let the muscles in your back relax when you drop your spine down into the sway-back position. Counting both movements as one repetition, do several repetitions.

4. Stand erect and raise your straight arms overhead, first from the side and then from the front. Do about four repetitions in each direction, breathing "in" as you lift your arms.

5. Lock your fingers behind your head and lean backward slightly as you lift your chest and move your head, shoulders, and elbows backward. Inhale as you lift your chest.

Summary

1. Basically, all lifting should be done by squatting down with the back flat (with both feet parallel and flat on the floor) and then lifting with the legs. Keep your spine as vertical as possible, and stand close to the object you are lifting.

2. When you are supporting or carrying a heavy object, always let it rest against your body.

3. When you have to push a large object, lean against the object with your arms bent so that you can put your body-weight into the effort. Keep your back flat and drive with your legs.

4. The technique of pulling is similar to that of pushing, except that you lean away from the object you are pulling so that the driving force of your legs is in line with a straight spine.

5. One of the main causes of backache in industry stems from prolonged static postures (sitting or standing) that do not permit enough movement to relieve tension on the muscles and joints. For this reason, it is a good idea to take a mid-morning and mid-afternoon "exercise break" (such as the one described in this chapter) in order to relieve stiffness and to restore circulation.

11

What to Do About
"Nervous Backache"

A great many people have backache for which there is no apparent physical cause, and they are usually told by their doctors that their trouble is "just your nerves." It is true, of course, that many backaches are caused by "nerves," but considering all of the things that can go wrong in the tremendously complicated and hidden structures of the back and spine, it is rarely wise to take it for granted that your back trouble is being caused by your nerves until a complete examination has been made. Since unrelieved backache can cause nervousness, it is sometimes difficult to tell which comes first, the nervousness or the backache. For this reason, a search should always be made for structural causes of backache before attention is centered on the nervous system.

Probable Sources of "Nervous" Backache

As you learned in other chapters of this book, simple tension and strain on the muscles, joints, and ligaments from weak muscles, poor posture, improper lifting techniques, or bad working conditions can cause backache that may range from a vague discomfort to acute distress. Back muscles can become chronically inflamed from exposure, systemic disorders, and other disturbances that may not be obvious or detectable on the surface.

Thus, there are a great many things that can cause backache, and your doctor must systematically eliminate them before labeling your backache as "nerves." *Furthermore, anyone who has a backache should make a special effort to correct any physical disorder or indiscretion (according to the procedures outlined in this book) that might be a cause of backache, regardless of the condition of the nervous system.*

A nervous backache is nothing to be ashamed of, however, and it is just as real and painful as a nervous person's stomach ulcers. Medical science has known for a long time that nervous tension could spill over from the brain into the various organs and structures of the body. But for some reason not yet clear to medical sleuths, disturbed and excessive psychic energy may affect each person differently. One man, for example, might develop stomach ulcers, while another might suffer from "tension headaches." And there are a large number of other disorders (such as colitis, asthma, skin ailments, indigestion, and so on) that are believed to occur as a direct result of nervous stress. In fact, there is hardly an organ in the body that cannot be affected adversely or psychosomatically in a functional way by a flooding storm of nervous tension.

We all remember the news releases on the work of Dr. Hans Selye, the medical researcher who found that the stress and strain of living in today's highly competitive society causes nervous and hormone imbalances which result in many chronic and seemingly incurable diseases.

Do not set your sights too high in this unstable world of ours, and do not take on more work than you can handle. People who worry constantly in efforts to meet impossible deadlines are bound to get sick. You can get ahead by taking one step at a time, and you can live for each day as it comes.

What Causes "Nervous" Backache?

Since the structures of the back are not as directly connected to the involuntary nerve centers of the brain as the organs are, your chances of developing a nervous backache are less than your chances of experiencing a "lump" in your throat, an upset stomach, a palpitating heart, clammy hands, or some other signal indication of nervous tension. But "nerves" *can* cause backache, especially when the tension is expressed in tightened muscles. Chronic or prolonged nervous tension, for example, can cause muscular inflammation and spasm from continuous muscular tension. And in a way not yet fully understood by medical science, acute backache can develop in persons who suddenly come face to face with disaster, failure, or humiliation. All of the fear, pain, and anxiety generated by an agitated brain just seems to spill over into the nerve endings in the muscles of the back to cause a phantom-like pain that eludes detection.

I have seen many backaches caused by nervous tension, and once the nature of a nervous person's backache becomes obvious, his trouble can usually be associated with the recurring stresses and disappointments of life. I knew a service station operator, for example, who developed a variety of symptoms along with backache every time business was bad. And when he came in one day with a bad backache that was overshadowed by symptoms of anxiety, he did not have to tell me that he had lost his business to his creditors.

One of the most common disorders I see in my office is spasm or inflammation of the muscles on the back of the neck from severe or prolonged tension. We have all experienced the tightness that seems to grip our neck and throat when we are under a great deal of tension. When this tension is prolonged, a waste product released by the taut muscles causes inflammation which can cause painful neck-locking muscle spasm. I have a number of patients who work under such great pressure that nervous tension is a constant problem, and when they begin to feel their neck tightening up, they return for relaxing manipulation.

One of the worst stiff necks I have ever seen occurred in a man who hated his job and who could not make up his mind about going into business for himself. He had a fairly large family and was barely able to support them on the salary he was making, but so much risk was associated with the new business venture he had in mind that he suffered two years of indecision and stiff neck. When he finally did make the change and was successful, his neck trouble disappeared.

Marital problems, business pressures, a nagging mate, meddling in-laws, a problem child, and other common aggravations of life can cause backache. It has been my observation that marital problems are a big cause of nervous backache in women. In many cases, a thoughtless husband who fails to attend to the needs of his wife with patience, tenderness, and affection is to blame. At other times of course the wife is at fault.

When husbands or wives complain to me about the actions of a mate, I usually tell them that if they will be patient and kind and sincerely try to please each other, things will work out. Nothing cuts deeper into love than words, and when that first word is spoken in anger or vengeance about something so sensitively balanced as marital love, wounds are opened that may never heal if they are not received with patience and forgiveness.

I have also seen backache develop in older people when their married children ignored them on various occasions.

Many people who have nervous backache become aware of the nature of their trouble when backache repeatedly follows a family squabble, a failure to make a sale, or some other highly distressing or unnerving experience. In some cases, nervous fatigue or backache results as an excuse for failure or because of a fear of responsibility, and it is fabricated by the subconscious mind as a defense reaction to "save face." Most of the time, such backache will be accompanied by other symptoms, such as an excessive amount of "gas," difficulty in swallowing, excessive perspiration in some part of the body, inability to rest or sleep, headache, inability to meet people, difficulty in breathing, depression, and so on.

Needless to say, persons who have personal, mental, and emotional problems that are causing backache must make an effort to face up to or correct their problems. In some cases, for example, this may mean that an individual must either change his attitude or change his circumstances.

Many people who harbor gripes and resentments can get rid of their backache by expressing themselves forcefully. Some may have to empty their hostilities into athletic activities. Others can work off their frustrations and tensions in love, hobbies, or exercise. Highstrung persons who simply have too much nervous energy to relax can prevent the development of backache tension by channeling their energy into such constructive activities as art, photography, physical training, or writing. Many unhappy people who are burdened with insurmountable problems can keep tension from building up by participating in helpful and constructive work that will take their mind off their worries.

If you have more than your share of problems, the important thing is to understand the nature of your situation and then try to meet the challenge of correcting it or making the most of it! If an inmate of Alcatraz can become a world-famous authority on bird diseases (it really happened!), you certainly ought to be able to live a happy, helpful, and constructive life in a free society. If you feel that you cannot make it alone, do not hesitate to see a psychiatrist for a little help.

Unhealthy living can also be a cause of nervous fatigue, which can cause backache. No one who eats improperly, sleeps irregularly, or works excessively should expect to be able to keep going without experiencing backache or exhaustion.

Exercise to Work off Nervous Tension

When you have a nervous backache that is not related to organic changes or that cannot be corrected by a simple change in attitude or circumstances, you might find exercise to be most effective in relieving your symptoms. And since so many "nervous backaches" are really physical in nature, and since nervous energy can best be worked off in physical exercise, many people will find that the improvement in posture and muscle tone resulting from exercise will eliminate many undetected causes of backache.

Any kind of exercise (such as swimming, bicycle riding, running, walking, or handball) that will stimulate the circulation of blood and produce a mild fatigue would be effective in relieving nervous tension. But if you have a "nervous backache" that may or may not be caused by nervous tension, I would suggest that you do the exercises described in this book so that you can strengthen your back as you work off your tension, thus eliminating two possible causes of your back trouble.

The application of heat and massage, as recommended in Chapter 7, would also be of value in relieving the tension of nervous backache.

The Difference Between Fatigue and Tension!

If you perform heavy physical work, or if you have not been getting adequate rest or sleep, you may develop a type of physical and nervous fatigue in which sheer exhaustion makes your hand tremble and your back ache. When this is the case, you need rest and sleep rather than exercise. (See "The Backache of Overexertion" in Chapter 8.)

Obviously, you will have to use a little common sense in balancing your rest and exercise for a healthy nervous system.

People who wear themselves out from overwork or excessive worrying sometimes suffer from a form of nervous exhaustion called "neurasthenia," which could be the first step toward a nervous breakdown if the tension is not relieved.

How To Eliminate the Causes of Your Tension

In a great many cases, the backache of nervous tension will be labeled "fibrositis," "lumbago," or "rheumatism" by your doctor. Although any of the popular treatments for these disorders may temporarily relieve the symptoms, *they cannot remove the causes of your tension.*

Be honest with yourself. If personal and emotional problems are not recognized and corrected, your backache will go on and on, and your journey from one doctor to another in seeking the "true cause" of your backache might eventually lead you to a "doctor" who can "cure" you if you are able to pay a large sum of money in advance for a large number of "treatments."

Massage and manipulation at the hands of a competent chiropractor or osteopath can be very effective in relieving physical symptoms resulting from nervous tension that binds the muscles and joints, but if you become convinced that your trouble is being caused by some of your vertebrae being out of place, your failure to face reality and solve your problems at their roots (along with a constant fear of the position of your vertebrae) may create new and imaginary illnesses, and you may become a "vertebral cripple."

How to Relax

Anyone who has ever had medical care for a "nervous back-ache" has been told to "relax." But this is much easier to say than to do when no specific instructions are offered.

One of the best ways to relax when you are suffering from nervous tension is to simply make a change in your daily routine. At the end of each day, for example, you should participate in some kind of play or activity that you enjoy doing and that is completely different from what you have been doing all day long. If you do not want to indulge in simple exercise, you can play ball with the kids, work in the yard, or go for a swim, and so on—anything as long as you get out of the rut you are in from day to day! I know of a busy surgeon who races high-powered speed boats in national competition because he says that it is so different from the type of work he does everyday that it "re-laxes" him. I know a dentist who camps out on hunting trips on weekends, regardless of the weather, and comes back "refreshed."

Persons who are nervous and tense must make a special effort, several times a day, to relax both mind and body completely. It is believed, for example, that there is a close relationship between the state of the mind and the tension of the muscles! A nervous person who does not find ways to relax his muscles becomes more nervous, while a person who would not normally be nervous could develop symptoms of nervous tension if he allowed muscular tension to go unbroken each day. Thus, *when time is taken to relax the muscles, the mind relaxes when the muscles relax, and vice versa.* Furthermore, physiologists believe that there may be some connection between the tension of the muscles and the sleep centers of the brain; that is, when the muscles relax, the sleep centers of the brain are free to function. For this reason, persons who have trouble sleeping at night should first make an effort to secure muscular relaxation.

If you want a relaxing way to lie down for a short while, try lying on your back with a thin pillow under your head, a pillow under each knee, and a pillow under each arm (right next to your body).

Relaxing for Sleep

In many cases, sleep-inducing relaxation can be brought on

by light recreation or exercise which produces a mild fatigue. A warm bath, a good book, or a favorite television program might also help.

Unfortunately, many people have acquired the very bad habit of trying to *force* themselves to sleep. As a result, they literally tense up their muscles without realizing it in efforts to assume restful sleeping postures. They may close their eyes tightly, for example, or they may hold their head in a certain position with a considerable amount of tension up and down the muscles of their spine. And they wait in anticipation of sleep they hope will carry them off to dreamland on a magic mattress.

Check your own muscles when you retire tonight. Are you jamming your head back into your pillow? Are you squeezing your eye lids together? Are your arms drawn up tightly against your body? Are your hands clenched?

Most of the time, your muscles will be tense without your realizing it. For this reason, it may be necessary for you to tense your muscles and then relax them in order for you to tell whether you are tense or relaxed.

Just to make sure that tight muscles are not short-circuiting the sleep centers of your brain, try this muscle-relaxing technique: Pick each part of your body up from the mattress (one part at a time, of course) and then drop it. Let your muscles relax so that the body part will drop without resistance. Start with your head, for example, and let it drop back against your pillow. Next lift an arm up and let it fall. Do the same thing with your other arm, your lower back, and each leg. Try to relax completely so that the lifted body part will fall like a rock. It will take practice to be able to relax so completely, but once you develop such control you will be able to relax at will.

When you are trying to relax, visualize your muscles relaxing like a wilted flower. Let your muscles—especially your face muscles—sag. As your muscles relax, the reciprocal action of the sleep centers in your brain will promote further relaxation, which will in turn promote sleep. The concentration required to lift and drop your arms or legs will erase other thoughts from your mind, and as your muscles relax, your thought processes will slow down until the day's worries fade away.

Try to go to bed at the same time each night so that your body and mind will become conditioned for regular sleeping hours.

You will sleep better if your sleep becomes a timed habit that can be triggered by your subconscious mind each night.

RELAXING ON THE JOB

Even when you are on the job during the day, you should occasionally relax your muscles by letting them sag lifelessly for several seconds at a time. Do not let your tension build up to such an extent that your muscles grip your bones like over-stretched rubber bands. If you allow this to happen, you may become a victim of that vicious cycle of tension that exhausts the nerves, inflames the muscles, and dulls the mind—and you may carry it to bed with you each night. When you find physical and nervous tension creeping up on you, take a rest break and relax your muscles completely.

Do not schedule more to do each day than you can do without rushing around at a frantic pace. Once tension backache develops from over-stimulated and over-tensed muscles, bad habits and muscle inflammation make it impossible to get rid of your tension overnight.

SIX RULES FOR INSOMNIACS

If you suffer from insomnia in spite of your efforts to slow down and relax, there may be other reasons for your inability to sleep. Evening exercise, for example, tends to promote sleep by producing mild fatigue, but if indulged in too strenuously just before bedtime it can key up the nervous system to such an extent that your senses are "wide awake" for hours after you go to bed. Excessive eating before bedtime can also cause insomnia, even though a light meal tends to promote sleep by diverting blood from the brain to the stomach. Coffee or tea before bedtime is another common cause of inability to sleep.

If you read yourself to sleep each night, you might be able to speed things along by doing your reading in a sitting position so that the pull of gravity will reduce the flow of blood to your brain.

If you are an insomniac, follow these simple rules:

1. Establish regular sleeping hours and stick to them. Do not sleep late or take an afternoon nap, even though you "did

not sleep the night before." You should not expect to sleep at night if you take naps during the day.

2. When your work ends for the day, do not take your job worries home with you. Avoid "homework" that requires heavy concentration before bedtime, lest your over-stimulated brain keeps clicking after you go to bed.

3. Try to cultivate a mild physical fatigue by participating in light exercise or recreation each day before supper. But do not exercise after supper or just before bedtime.

4. Do not eat so much at night that you are uncomfortable, and do not drink coffee or tea before bedtime. Coffee contains caffein and tea contains theine, and both of these substances are nervous system stimulants which can cause sleeplessness. Furthermore, both tea and coffee contain tannic acid which retards digestion and produces constipation, thus adding another barrier to restful sleep. Even cocoa contains a substance called "theobromine," which is a mild stimulant, and it also contains a small amount of tannic acid. Cola drinks are stimulating enough to interfere with the sleep of some people, so it might be a good idea to stick to milk or fruit juice for evening beverages.

5. Make sure that your bedroom is well ventilated, dark, and quiet—and try to keep the room temperature comfortable. When a room is hot and stuffy it is impossible to rest completely.

6. If you still have trouble sleeping, take a warm bath and then sit in a comfortable reclining chair with your head back and your eyes closed until you begin to doze; then crawl into a nearby bed that has already been prepared for sleeping.

If you can relax during the day and then get a good night's sleep, you should be able to overcome or prevent nervous backache.

Summary

1. Although "nerves" are a common cause of backache, many backaches that are labeled "nervous backaches" have hidden physical causes that can be erased with proper attention to the use of exercise and good posture.

2. When nervous backache does occur, however, it is just as real and uncomfortable as any other kind of backache. And while the physical symptoms of such a backache can be relieved by exercise, massage, manipulation, and other forms of physical treatment, it cannot be cured unless the underlying mental or emotional causes are removed.

3. Because of the reciprocal action between the muscles and the sleep centers of the brain, techniques that are effective in relaxing the muscles at night will also promote sleep. (See "Relaxing for Sleep" at the end of this chapter.) You can also lessen nervous tension by relaxing your muscles, and you can avoid prolonged muscular tension by keeping your nervous tension broken with hobbies, exercise, and recreation.

4. It is important to have regular sleeping hours and to get adequate sleep each night. Exercise or recreation that will produce a mild fatigue before sitting down for a light supper, followed by a warm bath and an hour or so of reading in a sitting position, should make it easier to fall off to sleep. (See the "Six Rules for Insomniacs" at the end of this chapter.)

5. The pressures of everyday living can cause backache if you do not learn to relax and to take things as they come.

6. Remember that it is just as important to prevent nervous backache as it is to prevent back strain; so even if you are not suffering from nervous tension at the present time, you should follow the instructions offered in this chapter in order to *prevent* the development of such symptoms.

12

Specific Exercises for Prevention and Correction of Backache

If your backache is not alleviated by avoiding stresses caused by bad posture, improper working conditions, incorrect lifting techniques, or emotional tension, then it is a safe assumption that you need to take a little regular exercise to correct the cause of your backache—that is, of course, if your doctor has found nothing seriously wrong with your back.

TEST YOURSELF WITH THESE FIVE PRELIMINARY EXERCISES

Although everyone can benefit from exercises that are designed to increase strength and flexibility, there are some people who are weaker or stiffer than others and who are likely candidates for a serious or painful back injury if they do not take immediate steps to correct their weaknesses. Test yourself with these simple exercises and see if you have physical liabilities that might contribute to the development of backache.

165

1. Lie flat on your back and slowly raise one straight leg up *past* a 45 degree angle while the opposite leg is flat against the floor. If a painful pulling sensation behind your knee prevents you from completing the exercise, the tendons on the back of your leg are too tight and you have lost your flexibility, which can be a cause of backache (See Figure 12).

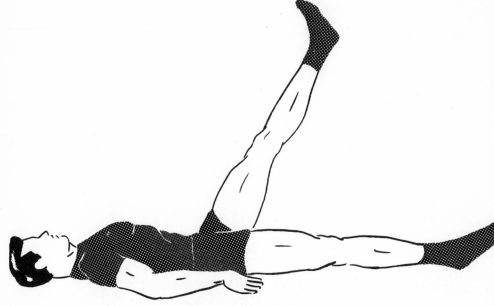

Figure 12:   Test exercise 1

2. Lie face down over a padded chair with your pelvis supported by the chair seat. Support the upper half of your body by placing your hands on the floor. Then put your hands behind your head and see if you can hold your back straight while someone holds your legs down. If you cannot hold this position for 6 seconds, your back muscles are too weak to offer adequate protection for your spine (See Figure 13).
3. Raise both legs up straight while you are lying flat on your back. If you cannot complete the exercise, or if you must strain to do it, your hip flexors are too weak to provide balanced support for your spine on its front side (See Figure 14).

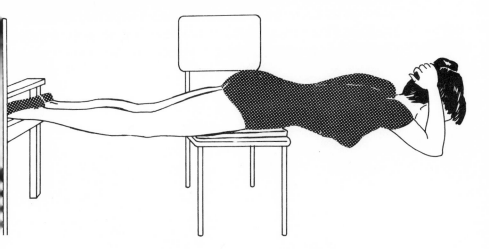

Figure 13: Test exercise 2

Figure 14: Test exercise 3

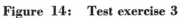

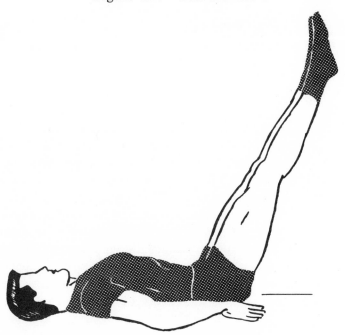

4. Do a bent-knee situp with your feet anchored and your hands behind your head. If you cannot do the exercise without starting off with a jerk, your abdominal muscles are too weak to maintain the best posture (See Figure 15).

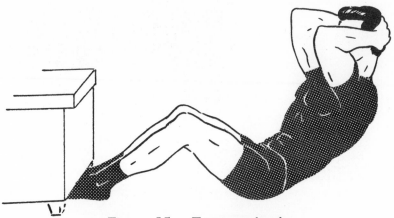

Figure 15: Test exercise 4

5. Do a full squat on your toes with your hands on your hips and your spine straight up and down. If you cannot complete the squat without leaning forward, bouncing, or "crawling up your thighs" with your hands, your thigh muscles are too weak to use in correct lifting techniques (See Figure 16).

WEAK MUSCLES ARE A COMMON CAUSE OF BACKACHE

You have already learned that a common factor underlying chronic backache is lack of sufficient support from muscles that are too flabby and too weak to protect the spinal joints when the back is under stress. And when the back muscles are weak, even the pull of gravity causes the joints to sag and strain against their ligaments. For this reason, exercise should be an important part of your effort to *prevent* backache. If you failed any of the test exercises, you should concentrate on similar exercises described in this chapter, but the body as a whole—not just the back—should be strengthened if maximum protection for the back and spine is to be obtained. Weak legs or arms, for example, would result in considerably more strain being placed upon the spine during

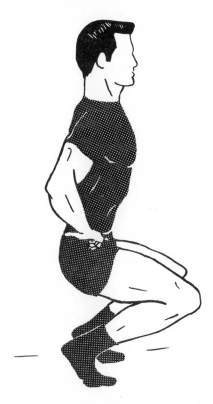

Figure 16: Test exercise 5

heavy lifting, since the muscles of the back would be compelled to assume most of the load.

In any event, there are many muscles in the arms, neck, hips, and thighs that overlap and support the action of certain muscles in the back. Muscles in the thighs and hips, for example, are important in low-back support, and they aid in forward and backward bending of the spine. Certain muscles in the shoulders and upper arms attach to structures in the back, thus acting very much like back muscles. Even the abdominal muscles provide important support for the spine on its front side.

In the exercises to be described in this chapter, emphasis will be placed upon development of muscles that are directly concerned with supporting the spine in an upright position, but many other important and overlapping exercises will be described in order to assure all-round strength and development, thus providing maximum protection for the spine. And in order to make sure that your development is balanced and even on both sides of your body for correction and prevention of spinal curvatures, no one-armed or one-legged exercises that affect the trunk in a lopsided manner have been described. All of the exercises are safe and simple, and all are designed to aid postural reflexes, but *do not do any of the exercises that cause pain or discomfort.*

Be careful not to exercise too much or too often. I have been exercising most of my life (and enjoying it!), and my articles on physical training appear regularly in various physical training magazines and journals. So I speak from experience when I say that exercising three times a week (every other day) is adequate for developing and strengthening the muscles if you are not an athlete training for competition. You will become stale and bored with your exercises if you do them everyday. So try to stick to the every-other-day routine when it is convenient, no matter how enthusiastic you might become about your exercises, and do not do more exercise than recommended.

When you do not have time to do the recommended number of repetitions for maintaining muscular strength, try to do each exercise a couple of times through a full range of movement in order to maintain your flexibility.

WHY SHOULD YOU EXERCISE?

If you are seriously interested in preventing backache, you should exercise for a number of reasons.

Well-toned back muscles make it easier to stand and sit erect without fatigue, and there is less chance of straining the back and spine in unaccustomed efforts. Furthermore, proper exercises will prevent the muscle-shortening that pulls the spine out of alignment to create a constant backache from loss of flexibility and balance. Regular exercise will also prevent the formation of irritating "muscle deposits" that trigger recurring muscle spasms.

Here are the muscle findings in the case history of a female patient who had chronic backache from lack of exercise.

How a Housewife Rid Herself of Backache

Mrs. Alice B., a 36-year-old housewife with 3 children, had suffered from backache since the birth of her first child 15 years ago. And on a number of occasions, she was incapacitated by such severe muscle spasm and back pain that doctors thought that she might have a "slipped disc." X-ray and neurological examination was always negative, however, and she was usually dismissed with a diagnosis of "back strain" or "possible disc trouble." She was treated with traction, manipulation, back supports, heat, injections, and many other types of treatment used and recommended by a number of different doctors. She got some relief from such treatment, but her trouble always returned, and she continued to have frequent "back spasms." A few doctors suggested that she take a little exercise, but most of them recommended rest; so Alice rested, as she had been doing for the past 15 years.

Physical examination revealed a typical sedentary posture. She was sway-backed and round-backed, and she had a perfectly round and prominent "pot belly" below her navel. Her head was thrust forward like a chicken, and her chest was flat. Her thighs and buttocks were flabby and shapeless, and she was too weak to do a full squat without climbing up her legs with her hands. There were a number of tender spots in the muscles around her lower back and hips. Her abdominal muscles and hip flexors were too weak to do a single two-legged straight-leg raise while lying on her back, and she found simple situps impossible to do. In addition, she had very little flexibility, and the muscles on the back of her legs were so tight that she could not reach any further than 6 inches below her knee caps while standing with her legs straight.

I recommended several of the exercises described in this chapter for Alice B. I demonstrated each exercise for her and then sketched them on a sheet of paper and gave it to her so that she would not forget what to do. After six weeks she was "feeling much better." After three months her backache was "about gone," and her physical appearance was 100 percent improved. When I saw her at the end of six months, *she had no backache at all* and she was much more attractive physically.

Men, of course, can suffer from the same type of backache that plagued Alice B., and their physical appearance can be just as bad. Any man or woman who gets no exercise at work or play should take a little regular exercise at home, whether backache is a problem or not.

PROGRESSIVE EXERCISE WITHOUT APPARATUS

Since the greatest majority of people are compelled to exercise at home without apparatus of any kind, simple free-hand exercises which utilize the resistance of the bodyweight are usually most convenient. In any event, such exercises will adequately strengthen the muscles responsible for good posture, and they will increase the flexibility of the spine. Persons who find barbell exercises more convenient, or who want extraordinary muscular strength for added protection in heavy work or strenuous athletics, may begin the exercises in Chapter 13.

HOW TO BEGIN YOUR FREE-HAND EXERCISES

Do the exercises described at least three times a week, or on Monday, Wednesday, and Friday. Begin with only a few repetitions (three or four) and work up to the recommended number over a period of several weeks by progressively adding a few repetitions each week.

In increasing the amount of exercise you do, be guided by the amount of soreness or fatigue you experience. If you should "give out" or suffer from unusual muscle soreness following your exercises, it would be better to decrease the amount you do than to increase it. Severe or uncomfortable reactions to unaccustomed exercise can be avoided, however, if you will begin lightly and increase your exercise in a progressive manner as you become stronger and more flexible. Many people who claim that exercise gives them a backache are simply taking too much exercise or doing the wrong exercises. Regardless of what kind of exercise you do, you must begin gradually and lightly. And if you discontinue your exercise for two weeks or longer, you must again begin lightly. Do not be like the patient who takes a hard workout once or twice a month and then complains because the exercise makes him too sore to exercise more often.

When you first begin your exercises, you may discover that you are "stiff" in some portions of your body. You will, of course, have to loosen up these areas by concentrating on the exercises that reveal the stiffness, but do not try to do it all at once by doing your exercises forcefully. You can become extremely sore by overstretching a tight muscle. So be cautious.

In order to strengthen your back without straining it, your exercises should be fairly comfortable to perform. If you find any of the basic exercises in this book too difficult to do, there may be a modified version of the exercise (in the same group) that you can do to prepare you for the more difficult exercise. If you will just follow the instructions accompanying the exercises, you will not be straining in your exercises.

It will usually take two or three weeks of regular, light exercise before you will be able to indulge in moderately heavy exercise without experiencing extreme muscle soreness or lameness. And it may take several weeks of regular exercise to show much visible improvement. But the benefits to be obtained from a few minutes of exercise three times a week are so great that you cannot afford to pass up such an investment.

It has been my experience that once the muscles have been strengthened by regular exercise, they can be kept strong by short twice-a-week workouts when time is at a premium. This observation has been substantiated in the research of Dr. Richard Berger of Texas Technological College.

Always warm up before making a maximum effort in any exercise. You can do this by doing a few repetitions of the exercise you are about to do and then resting a few minutes before doing a full set (as many repetitions as you can do). Preliminary warmup exercise increases the flow of blood to the exercised muscles, thus warming up the fibers and decreasing the possibilities of muscle strain. An increased blood flow will also provide a better supply of the chemical substances necessary for muscular contraction. And a minute or two of rest between exercises will permit the fresh, oxygen-filled blood to oxidize waste products and replenish energy stores for the next exercise.

Try to exercise at a time when your mind is free from distracting worries. You can get more benefit from your exercises and you will use more muscle fibers if you can concentrate on what you are doing. As a general rule, it is usually best to exercise about two hours before or after a meal. Most people will prefer to exercise before supper.

The exercises marked with an asterisk are considered to be the most important for strengthening the muscles directly concerned with supporting the spine. If you do not want to do one or more of the exercises in each group, you should at least do one exercise from each of the asterisk-marked groups.

Many of the exercises in the various groups are designed for stronger or weaker persons, so be sure to read the instructions accompanying each exercise before you do it. You may alternate similar exercises for variety and for fun if you like.

How to Breathe During Your Exercises

Try not to hold your breath during any of your exercises, especially during squats, situps, and leg raises. When you take a deep breath and hold it during an exertion, the pressure created in your chest and abdomen might interfere with the flow of venous blood back to your heart, which could result in excessive fatigue or dizziness from a diminished flow of blood to your brain.

Breathe rhythmically during your exercises, and exhale during exertion; that is, breathe "out" when muscular contraction seems to tighten up the chest or abdomen, and "in" when muscular relaxation permits expansion of the rib cage. When you are not sure how to breathe in an exercise, just breathe anyway that is most convenient for you—as long as your breathing is regular and rhythmical.

(Group 1) "Back-Limbering" Bending Exercises

Bending exercises are designed more for developing and maintaining flexibility than for muscular development. Try to do all of the exercises in this group.

(A) *Side bending:* With your hands on your hips, bend from side to side 10 to 12 times. Perform the exercise smoothly with a moderate speed. Fast or forceful bending might result in a ligamentous strain, or it might disturb a weak or defective joint (See Figure 17).

(B) *Forward bending:* Bend forward (letting your spine bend) and touch your toes 8 to 10 times. If you find it difficult or impossible to reach your toes, stop the bending when discomfort occurs. It is not really necessary to actually touch your toes

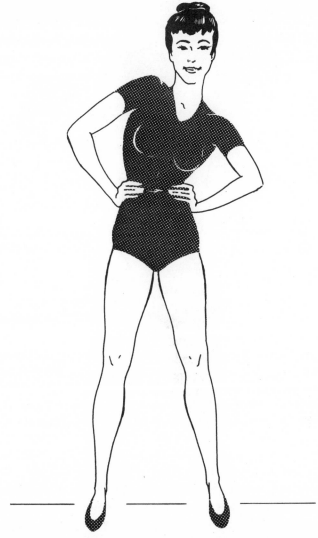

Figure 17: Side bending. Exercise "A" of Group 1

in this exercise. The more flexible you become, however, the farther forward you can bend (See Figure 18).

In any event, *do not use sudden or forceful movement in an
attempt to reach your toes in a toe-touching exercise.* Tight hamstrings on the back of your legs might tear or cause a torsion
strain to be transmitted to your pelvis, which might result in a

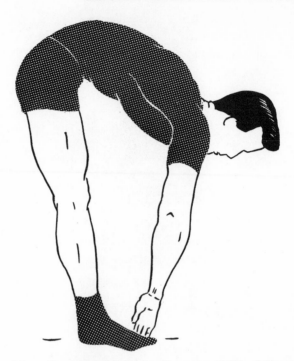

Figure 18:   Forward bending. Exercise "B" of Group 1

sacroiliac strain. Since tight hamstrings can be a cause of backache, it is usually a good idea to stretch them with special exercises, but it must be done gradually and without force. There
are some people whose bony structure will not permit them to
touch their toes under any circumstances, and it might be harmful for them to try to do so forcefully.

If you have a history of "slipped disc," you should keep your
back *flat* and your legs straight during forward bending exercises
(with your hands on your hips) so that all of the bending will
take place in your hip joints, thus stretching your hamstrings
without putting a compression strain on your spinal discs.

(C) *Twisting exercise:* Lie on your back with your trunk,
thighs, and legs flexed at right angles to each other, as though you
were sitting in an over-turned chair. Hold your legs in this "sitting position" and drop them first to one side and then to the
other side by twisting at your waist. Keep your shoulders and
upper back flat on the floor, and place your arms along side your
body with your hands palms-down on the floor for counterbal-

ance. Do several repetitions in each direction. This exercise will maintain rotary flexibility in your spine, and it will keep your vertebrae properly adjusted (See Figure 19).

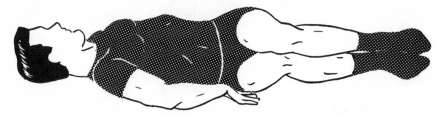

Figure 19: Twisting exercise. Exercise "C" of Group 1

Twisting exercises in an erect standing or sitting position should be avoided because of the strain they place on the knees and the sacroiliac joints. If you twist while standing, for example, you might twist a knee joint, since your anchored lower leg cannot turn with the rest of your body (twist dancers, beware!); and if you twist while sitting, you might strain a sacroiliac joint because of your pelvis' being anchored on the chair seat.

(D) *Backward bending:* Backward bending or "hyperextension" of the spine in a standing position is not a safe exercise for most people, especially when there is a history of back trouble. It would be best, as a general rule, for everyone to avoid any kind of backward bending that is uncomfortable and do only the back-arching exercise described below in Group 2.

However, if you sit or stand all day, you might be able to relieve some of the binding fatigue in your spinal joints by sitting in a chair that has a low back, and then leaning backward.

(Group 2) "Back-Straightening" Back-Arching Exercises *

Exercise "A" of this group is one of the exercises most often prescribed by orthopedic specialists for toning up and developing the muscles up and down the spine. Since hyperextension of the spine in this exercise can be carried only as far as normal muscular contraction will permit, there is no danger of ligamentous strain, as there is in backward bending while standing.

If you are extremely sway-backed, or if you experience some discomfort in back-arching exercises, you can strengthen the same

---

* Important basic exercises.

muscles without backward bending by doing the barbell dead-lift exercise (number 7) described in Chapter 13.

(A) *Back arching from a flat surface:* Lie face down on a rug with a thick pillow under your pelvis. Anchor your feet by placing them under the edge of a heavy sofa or by having someone hold them down for you. Without using your arms to push up, raise the upper half of your body from the floor by arching your back. You do not have to arch up as high as you can. Stay well within a comfortable range of movement. Do this exercise eight to ten times (See Figure 20).

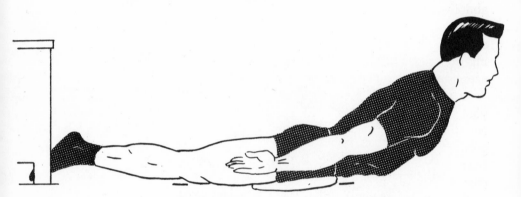

Figure 20: Back arching from a flat surface. Exercise "A" of Group 2

In addition to strengthening the spina erecta muscles, back-arching exercises, when done face-down with the feet anchored, will also strengthen the muscles on the back of the hips and thighs.

(B) *Back arching from a table:* This exercise is designed for those who find regular back arching easy and who want still stronger and larger spina erecta or back muscles.

Lying face down on a padded table with the upper half of the trunk hanging over the edge of the table and the lower half strapped to the table top (or anchored by the weight of a training partner), arch the upper body up from a low, hanging position; that is, start from a position in which the head is near the floor and then arch up. Do six to eight repetitions. In order to avoid pinching of the abdomen, the support of the table should end at the hips where most of the bending will take place.

(Group 3) "Stomach-In" Leg-Raising and Situp Exercises *

In maintaining good posture and a strong back, it is also important to keep the muscles on the front side of the spine in good condition. Like the guy wires of a TV broadcasting antenna, it takes the combined action of the muscles in front and the muscles in back to hold the spine erect. Well-developed abdominal muscles improve physical appearance by keeping the abdomen flat.

Exercise "A" of this group is another exercise frequently recommended by specialists who prescribe exercises for strengthening the spine. But if it causes you any discomfort, start out with exercise "B."

(A) *Straight leg raises:* Lie on your back with your arms at your sides and the palms of your hands flat on the floor for counterbalance. Keeping your legs straight, raise them up to a vertical position (straight up and down). Do not lower your legs back over your head; when gravity takes over, the movement ceases to be an abdominal exercise. Furthermore, forced flexion of the spine in jackknifing the body will place unnecessary strain on the spinal discs. Do as many leg raises as you comfortably can; 12 to 15 should be enough.

Leg raises develop the lower abdominal muscles and the muscles on the front of the thighs, as well as the deeper-lying hip flexors (iliopsoas muscles) that attach between the vertebrae in the lower part of the spine and the top of the thigh bones on each side. All of these muscles help support the spine on its front side.

If you cannot touch your toes in the forward bending exercise described earlier, or if straight leg raises seem to hurt your back, do one-legged straight-leg raises in order to stretch the tendons on the back of your legs. Keep one leg flat on the floor and raise the other leg (locked-out straight) as high as you can. Exercise both legs equally.

If you have a job in which you sit all day, work up to doing a few of your leg raises from the end of a low bench so that you can stretch your hip flexors. (When the hips stay flexed or bent all day in a sitting position, the muscles on the front of the hips may shorten enough to cause backache when you stand erect for long periods of time.) Lie down on the bench with your buttocks near the end of the bench, reach back over your head and grasp the bench with both hands, and then lower your straight legs until both heels touch the floor. If this puts an uncomfortable strain on your lower back, bend the knee of one leg and plant the foot of that leg flat on the floor while you raise and lower the opposite straight leg.

(B) *Knee-chest leg raises:* If you find straight-leg raises too difficult to do with both legs straight, or if they seem to hurt your lower back, you may bend your knees in your leg raises; that is, you start from a position with your legs flat on the floor and then bend your knees as you lift them up toward your chest. As you

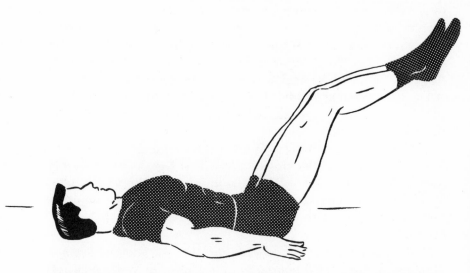

Figure 21: Knee-chest leg raises. Exercise "B" of Group 3

become stronger, however, you should try to gradually straighten out your legs until you can do straight-leg raises (See Figure 21).

Persons who do not have a history of "slipped disc," but who have leg pain being caused by a "pinched nerve" in the lower spine, might find relief from low-back discomfort and leg pain by lying on their side and pulling their knees up toward their chest until the lower back is rounded out, thus enlarging the openings between the vertebrae through which the nerves pass.

(C) *Situps:* Lying on your back with your hands behind your head, your knees *bent,* and your feet anchored, "sit up" by raising the upper half of your body from the floor. Do as many as you comfortably can (15 or 20 will be enough). In order to prevent irritation of the bony surfaces on the back of your pelvis, it will be necessary to put a thin cushion or a folded-up blanket under your hips as padding against the hard floor.

You can avoid excessive leverage on your lower spine, and place more work on the abdominal muscles, by making sure that you do your situps with your knees *bent;* otherwise, the deeper lying hip flexors, already exercised by the straight leg raises, will be forced to do most of the work.

Persons who are unusually weak or unable to do situps may do "trunk curls" in which the abdominal muscles are tightened up in lifting only the head and shoulders from the floor. (Actually, trunk curls alone would provide adequate exercise for the abdominal muscles, but since the hip flexors are also important in supporting the spine on its front side, an effort should be made to work up to full situps in which some bending takes place in the hips—especially if straight-leg raises are not being done.)

(D) *Frog kicks:* Hang from a high chinning bar, lift your knees up toward your chest (by bending your trunk, hips, and knees), and then lower your legs into a relaxed hanging position. If you will do this exercise correctly (that is, if you will lift your knees up as high as you can in a knee-chest position, and then relax your low-back muscles when you lower your legs), it will strengthen both your hip flexors and your abdominal muscles, *and it will stretch your spine and align your vertebrae* (See Figure 22).

(*Group 4*) Squatting Exercises for Correct Lifting Ability *

All of us are familiar with the safety rule stating that heavy lifting (or any lifting for that matter) should be done with the back straight, letting the legs do the actual lifting. Obviously,

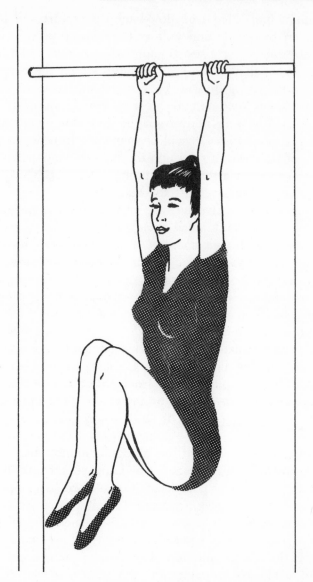

Figure 22:   Frog kicks. Exercise "D" of Group 3

the stronger your legs are, the less the chances are that you will strain your back.

Although squatting exercises are designed to strengthen the muscles of the thighs, they are also important for developing certain hip muscles that aid in supporting the lower back and in protecting the sacroiliac joints. There is no such thing as a strong back if the hips and thighs are weak and undeveloped.

Squatting exercises in high repetitions are also great for strengthening the heart and building physical fitness. According to a joint report released by the American Medical Association and the American Association for Health, Physical Education, and Recreation, exercise involving the use of the large muscles of the thighs is best for stimulating the movement of a large volume of blood—and "the oftener the normal heart and circulatory system are required to move blood to active regions of the body, the more efficient they become." The report also stated that the older we become, the more important it is to take a little regular exercise. So regardless of your age, you can strengthen both your back and your heart by following the exercises in this book; that is, of course, unless there is some medical reason why you cannot take exercise.

(A) *Flat-footed squat:* Starting from a standing position with your hands on your hips, squat down; keep your feet flat on the floor, putting your arms out in front for balance (as you squat) if necessary. See Figure 23.

If free squatting exercises seem too difficult to begin with, either because of poor balance or lack of strength, hold on to a bed post for aid or balance. Work up to 12 to 15 repetitions.

Squats may also be done with the heels on a board for easier balancing, but flat-footed squats are a better all-round exercise for strengthening muscles in both the hips and thighs simultaneously in cultivating correct lifting technique. Persons who have a hernia or some other abdominal disorder, however, should do squatting exercises with their heels on a thick board in order to keep the spine more vertical and to avoid compression of the abdomen. Half squats may be done to avoid excessive leverage on weak or injured knees.

There are many "healthy" people who cannot even do a full squat without climbing up their legs with their hands. Obviously, it would be impossible to keep the spine straight and vertical in correct lifting procedures if the thighs are too weak to even do a full squat.

In full-squat exercises, do not "bounce" at the bottom of the

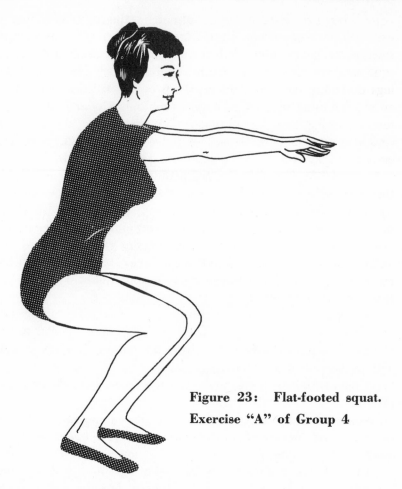

**Figure 23:   Flat-footed squat.
Exercise "A" of Group 4**

squat, lest you strain the ligaments in your knees. Do your squats smoothly and evenly. You may pause between squats while you are in a standing position, but you should not relax or pause at the bottom of the squat.

(B) *Half squatting from a chair:* Persons who are unable to do the squatting exercises described above can usually do this one with little or no trouble.

From a sitting position in a chair, stand up and return to your seat as many times as you comfortably can without pushing against your knees with your hands.

(C) *Leg-extension exercise:* This is a thigh exercise that is usually done only when knee trouble, back trouble, abdominal trouble, or some other disturbance makes it impossible to do squatting exercises in any manner. Sit on a high table with your legs dangling and your feet off the floor. Tie a weight (such as an old handbag filled with canned goods) to your foot and extend your leg to a straight, locked-out position. Use as much weight as you can for 10 correct repetitions. Exercise both legs equally.

Leg-extension exercises from a sitting position will not develop the muscles on the back of the thighs and hips as flat-footed squats will, but the back-arching exercises described earlier will provide adequate exercise for these muscles.

Keeping the thigh muscles strong during long periods of disabling back trouble will permit faster rehabilitation and protect the knees from strain by keeping the tendons over the knee joints tight and well developed.

(Group 5) "Chest-Out" Breathing Exercises

A deep, well-developed rib cage is important in good posture and in keeping the spine balanced and erect; for this reason, breathing exercises should be a part of every back-strengthening program.

Since you will be breathing heavily when you finish your squatting exercises, you should go immediately to your breathing exercises.

(A) *Stiff-arm pullovers from the floor:* Lie on your back with a sandbag held at arm's length over your chest. (A solid dumbbell in each hand would do fine.) Holding on to the bag with both hands, lower the bag back over your head with straight arms until the bag touches the floor. Breathe "in" deeply as the weight is being lowered, and then breathe "out" as you return the weight to starting position.

The chest muscles involved in this straight-arm pullover exercise will lift the chest high, and the forced deep breathing will expand the rib cage. (Certain back muscles are also activated.)

Use a weight that is light enough to permit 10 to 12 *easy* repetitions.

(B) *Stiff-arm pullovers from an ottoman:* After you become accustomed to doing pullovers on the floor, try doing them from the end of a low bench, or by lying back over an ottoman, for greater stretching of the rib cage; that is, of course, if you want a deeper chest for better-looking posture. See Figure 24.

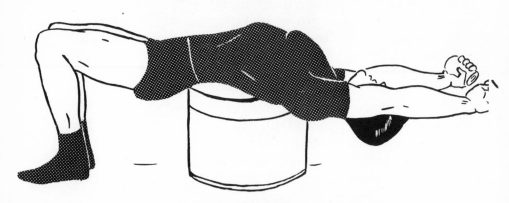

Figure 24: Stiff-arm pullovers from an ottoman. Exercise "B" of Group 5

If you use a bench, lie with your head at the end of the bench; but if you use an ottoman (padded foot stool), place it between your shoulder blades.

When you use an ottoman, you will have to support the lower half of your body by planting both feet on the floor, but the pressure of the ottoman in the upper portion of your back will provide a good spine-straightening exercise—especially if you have spinal arthritis or poor posture.

(Group 6) "Shoulders-Back" Shoulder Exercises for Tireless Posture *

The exercises in this group are important in preventing the sagging neck and shoulder pain so often experienced by office workers and sedentary persons who get very little exercise and maintain tiring postures day in and day out. Muscles should always be more than strong enough to overcome the constant pull of gravity and still maintain strength in reserve. Such a protective degree of strength must be acquired by performance of

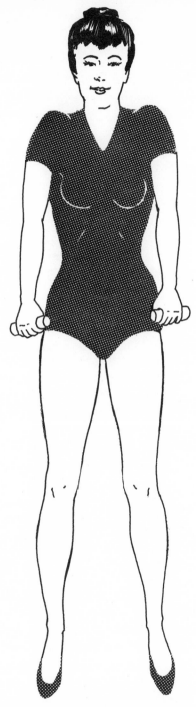

Figure 25: Shoulder shrugs. Exercise "A" of Group 6

exercises calling for full extension and contraction of the supporting muscles, preferably against resistance.

Except for the collar bones connecting the rib cage with the shoulder joints, only the muscles keep the bones of the arms, shoulders, and shoulder blades from sagging like a coat on a cloakroom hook.

(A) *Shoulder shrugs:* Since the trapezius and other muscles involved in supporting the shoulder girdle (from the neck to the tip of the shoulder) rarely receive adequate exercise in everyday activities, everyone should take special shoulder-shrugging exercises (See Figure 25).

Hold a sandbag or a dumbbell in each hand (down at arm's length at your sides) and "shrug" your shoulders by lifting them up toward your ears. Do 15 to 20 repetitions.

Strengthening the muscles of the shoulder girdle will help to prevent compression of nerves and blood vessels (that travel from the neck down into the arm) by a sagging collar bone.

(B) *Lateral shoulder raises:* Holding a can of beans or a dumbbell in each hand down at arm's length on each side, raise the weights from the sides, out, and overhead, keeping the arms straight. Ten to 12 repetitions should be adequate.

After a few minutes of rest, raise the weights forward and overhead several repetitions.

Both of these exercises will develop the deltoids and other muscles around and between the shoulders in back. See Figure 26.

(Group 7) Pushup Exercises

Pushup exercises are done primarily to develop the arms and chest, although certain muscles in the back are also brought into play. When the pectoral muscles of the chest, and the triceps muscles on the back of the arm, are strong, pushing movements that are so common in everyday activity can be done without bending or twisting the spine for "extra push."

(A) *Pushups:* This exercise is so well known that just about everyone knows how to do it, but there are many people who cannot do it correctly.

Lie face-down with your back straight and your feet together and "push up." Work up to 8 to 10 repetitions.

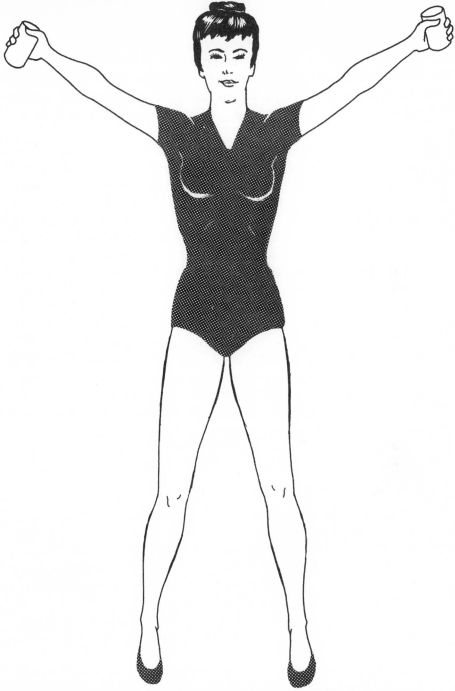

Figure 26: Lateral shoulder raises. Exercise "B" of Group 6

Men who want even greater strength and muscular girth can make the exercise a little harder (when regular pushups become easy) by doing it with both feet on a chair. The additional muscular effort required to keep the back straight during such exercise will further strengthen the spine.

(B) *Modified pushups:* This exercise is recommended for people, especially ladies, who are unable to do regular pushups.

Any exercise should be done several times to be of value, and when an individual can do only one or two repetitions there is more straining than training. Furthermore, better physical fitness, a stronger heart, and a slim waistline are best acquired by making sure that enough repetitions are done to result in increased breathing, a faster heart rate, and a little perspiration. For this reason, it is best to modify any exercise that is too difficult to do more than a few times. (Isometric exercise does not offer these benefits.)

To do modified pushups, lie face-down and "push up," keeping your back straight with your knees on the floor. Do as many repetitions as you comfortably can (See Figure 27).

As you become stronger, gradually change from the modified pushup to the regular pushup.

Figure 27:   Modified pushups. Exercise "B" of Group 7

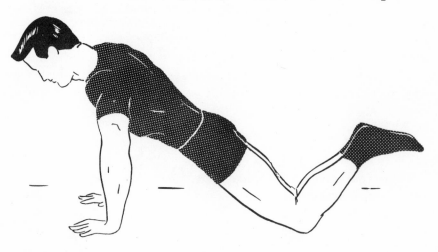

(Group 8) Chinning Exercises

Although most people think of chinning the bar as a bicep exercise, it is also a good back exercise. The latissimus dorsi muscles, for example, which give the upper back its wide "V"-shaped appearance, function in activities which call for pulling the arms down and back. There are many types of work in which the muscles developed by chinning will provide the extra "pulling strength" needed to protect the spine from strain during certain types of work and during emergencies.

(A) *Chinning the bar:* Grasp a horizontal bar with the palms of your hands facing away from you and "chin the bar." Work up to several repetitions. As a general rule, the bar should be just high enough for the individual to grasp while both feet are on the ground so that there will not be a fatiguing waste of energy in hanging from the bar between repetitions, and the hands should be placed about shoulder-width apart.

Chinning with the palms of your hands facing you will place more work on your biceps, while chinning with your palms facing away from you will place more work on the muscles of your back.

Try to install an adjustable chinning bar in the doorway of your bedroom for chinning and stretching exercises. Simply hanging from the bar a couple of times a day will give you a good spinal traction. You can easily make an adjustable horizontal bar by nailing slotted supporting blocks on the door-facing at selected levels so that you lift the bar up and place it at a desired level. (Some sporting goods stores sell doorway chinning bars.)

If chinning the bar is too difficult for you to do, that is, if you cannot do at least 2 or 3 repetitions, do the modified chins described below.

(B) *Modified chins:* This exercise is designed for ladies and other persons who find regular chins too difficult to do.

Place your doorway chinning bar (or a piece of iron pipe placed securely between two stepladders) at about chest level. Grasp the bar with your palms facing down. Then straighten-out your arms and your body, with your heels on the floor, so that you are hanging under the bar with your arms at a 90-degree angle to your body. Have someone brace your heels so they will not slip and then pull your body up and touch your chest to the bar. Do as many repetitions as you comfortably can. See Figure 28.

Figure 28: Modified chins. Exercise "B" of Group 8

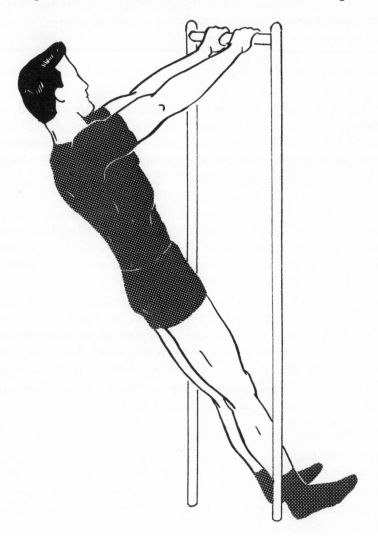

(Group 9) Stretching Tight Ankle Tendons

As you learned in an earlier chapter, abnormally short or tight hamstrings and ankle tendons can be a cause of backache, especially in women who habitually wear high-heeled shoes.

Exercise "B" in Group 1 of this chapter has already provided a means of stretching the hamstrings on the back of the thighs and knees. The exercises in this group will be concerned mainly with stretching the ankle tendons. (Most people who have short ankle tendons will not be able to lift their foot up to a position past a right angle to the lower leg while the leg is locked out straight.)

If you have reason to believe that your ankle tendons are too short, do both of the exercises in this group. (These exercises will also strengthen the feet and their arches for good foot posture, which will eliminate another possible cause of backache.)

(A) *The wall ankle stretch:* Standing flat-footed at arm's length from a wall (facing the wall), with both hands placed flat against the wall, lean forward by bending your arms. *Keep your heels on the floor, your toes pointed straight ahead, and your trunk straight.* Only your elbows, your shoulders, and your ankles bend in this exercise! Do 10 to 15 repetitions a couple of times a day (See Fig. 29).

(B) *Heel-lowering ankle stretch:* Stand on the edge of a step or a ledge with your weight supported on the front (ball) part of your feet. Lower your heels as far as you can in a heel raising and lowering exercise—that is, you rise up and down on your toes. Do only a few repetitions to begin with, lest the unaccustomed stretch makes your calves painfully sore, but work up to 15 to 20 repetitions over a period of time.

(Group 10) Test For Tight Thigh Bands

A less well-known but not uncommon cause of backache is found in tight (ilio-tibial) bands of tough connective tissue that run up and down the outside of each thigh. Persons who get no exercise at all and who sit all day will frequently suffer from thigh-band backache.

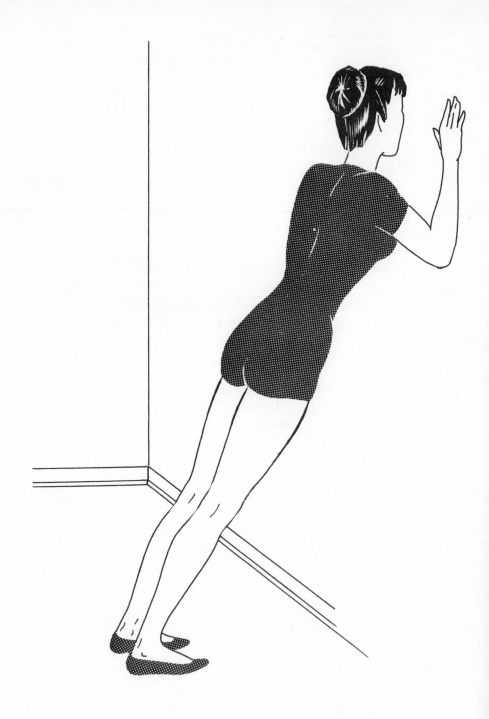

Figure 29:   The wall ankle stretch. Exercise "A" of Group 9

Try this test and see if you have tight thigh bands:

Lie on your side and pull the knee on the bottom side up toward your chest. Then bend the knee of the upper leg (placing your foot behind you) and move the leg backward. Relax and let the upper leg sag; if the knee will not drop down low enough to touch the floor, your thigh bands are too tight (See Figure 30).

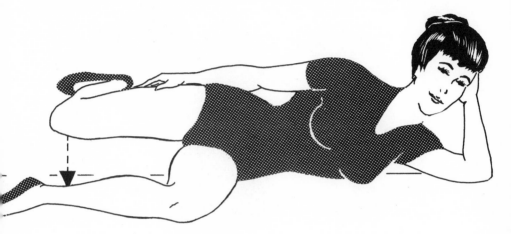

Figure 30:   Testing for tight thigh bands. Group 10

(A) *Stretching tight thigh bands:* Stand at arm's length from a wall, with the wall to your side. Place the palm of your extended arm (on the side next to the wall) against the wall and, by letting your arm bend, lean to that side by bending your legs sideways toward the wall. Keep your upper body straight and your beltline level with the floor so that all of the side bending will take place in your hips, thus stretching the outside of your thighs. Several repetitions on each side may be done about twice a day.

This exercise may also be done by placing your hand on the top of a high desk and then bending toward the desk. See Figure 31.

(Group 11) Your Neck as Possible Source of Backache

The neck is a common site of "back trouble," and it is probably one of the most neglected regions of the body when it comes

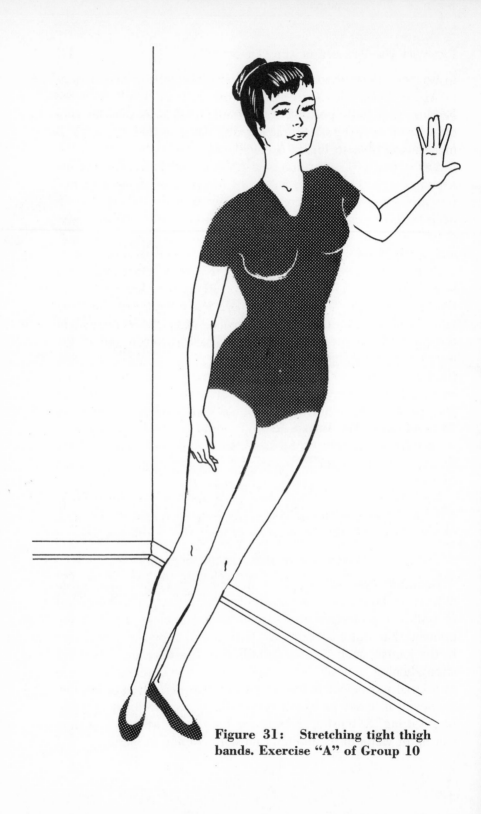

Figure 31: Stretching tight thigh bands. Exercise "A" of Group 10

to exercise. Furthermore, there are very few jobs or occupations in which the neck is required to do more than simply hold the head up in a static posture. As a result, weak neck muscles very often lead to "cricks," headache, and fatigue—and the neck is more susceptible to injury in accidents.

Almost without exception, the normal vertebral curve of the neck or cervical spine will flatten or reverse itself from a normal forward curve to an abnormal backward curve when a weak neck begins to cause trouble. For this reason, the neck exercises described in this group are designed to aid in restoring the normal curve of the neck as they increase muscular strength.

(A) *Neck exercise with a towel:* Tie a knot in each end of a large bath towel. Then tie one end of a long cord securely above the knot on one end of the towel, and make a loop on the other end of the cord so that you can loop it over the other end of the towel. With the cord fastened securely to each end of the towel, attach a weight to the middle of the cord and then drape the towel over your head like a bonnet. Exercise your neck by leaning forward and bracing your hands on your knees so that you can lift the weight up and down with your neck. Do 12 to 15 repetitions (See Figure 32).

(B) *Neck exercises by hand:* When you do not have the time to use a towel in your neck exercise, you can provide resistance by using your hands.

Lock your fingers behind your head and tilt your head backward as far as you can as you apply resistance against the back of your head. Do several repetitions a couple of times a day.

WHAT ABOUT ISOMETRIC EXERCISE?

Isometric exercise (working the muscles against immovable objects, without any movement in the joints) might be beneficial in building protective strength in back muscles, but it is my opinion that isotonic exercise (with a full range of movement in the joints), such as that described in this chapter, is best for strengthening a weak back, since restoration and maintenance of normal movement is the object in correction of back trouble. However, in cases in which very little joint movement is possible, "setting" or tensing the muscles for several seconds at a time can be of value in maintaining muscle size and strength.

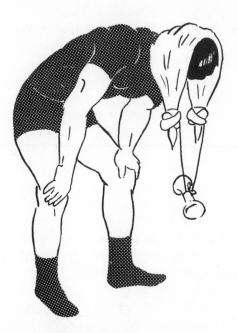

Figure 32: Neck exercise with a towel. Exercise "A" of Group 11

How to Exercise Your Back Isometrically

If you find yourself in bed and unable to stand erect for back exercises, there are at least two important isometric exercises that you can do to maintain muscle tone in the muscles supporting your lower back.

Lie face-down and tense your back muscles as though you were about to arch your upper body up from the bed. In other words, you only *begin* the back-arching exercise described in exercise "A" of Group 2 in this chapter—and you hold the beginning position for about 6 seconds.

Lie on your back with your knees bent and your feet flat on the mattress. Lift your feet up off the mattress a couple of inches and hold them there for several seconds.

Isometric exercises should be done three or four times a day for best results, especially if you are confined to bed.

Summary

1. If you fail any of the five test exercises described at the beginning of this chapter, concentrate on the exercises recommended for correcting the weakness or the stiffness uncovered by the test exercise. And if the test exercise in Group 10 reveals that you have tight thigh bands, include the exercise recommended for stretching the outside of your thighs.
2. In following the exercises in this chapter, begin with only three or four repetitions in each exercise and then gradually increase the amount of exercise you do over a period of time.
3. You should become accustomed to the exercises after doing them every other day for about three weeks, and you should be in fair shape with your back after about six weeks—and you should be feeling much better as well as looking much better.

   Remember that a small amount of prevention can save you from years of misery and treatment when it comes to back trouble.

13

General Barbell Exercises
for Strengthening the
Back Muscles

Although the exercises in Chapter 12 are best for preventing or correcting certain abnormalities in the spine, barbell exercises are probably more convenient and more effective for developing general all-round strength. And those who want considerable muscular strength for additional protection in heavy or strenuous activities can become stronger faster by taking simple barbell exercises. Furthermore, *barbell exercises train the back and the muscles to lift correctly and efficiently in activities which require heavy lifting.*

I had a good friend who, for financial reasons, was compelled to switch from a low-paying desk job to a job driving and loading freight trucks. When he told me about the pending change, I advised him to begin taking barbell exercises in order to strengthen his body in preparing for the new job if he wanted to protect his weak back from strain. He did not follow my advice, however, and when he strained his back for the third time after several weeks on the job, I told him that he had either better begin taking the exercises or start looking for a new job. So he started his barbell exercises, and he spent about 20 minutes doing squats (with 50 pounds), deadlifts (with 50 pounds), upright rowing motions (with 50 pounds) and bench presses (with 75 pounds) on Monday, Wednesday, and Friday. Within 6 weeks he had doubled the amount of weight he was using in his exercises, and after 3 months he was so strong that the freight he loaded caused little or no uncomfortable stress on his back.

You do not have to load freight trucks to benefit from strong back and body muscles, however. Just about everyone, at one time or another, will be forced to do a little heavy lifting. So it is best to be prepared for it.

I have seen many mothers experience back strain for the first time in lifting and carrying around a new baby. And when a woman is so weak that she can barely do an unaided full squat with her bodyweight alone, she will be compelled to lift with her back instead of with her legs when she lifts a baby from the floor.

Thus, anyone can benefit from light barbell exercises, and persons who must prepare for lifting tasks of any kind will find the exercises in this chapter more effective than the exercises in Chapter 12.

Barbell exercises are also very effective for correcting postural disorders in the upper back and shoulders where muscular support is so essential in supporting the spine and shoulder girdle. Because of the tension placed on nerves and muscles that pass down between the neck and the shoulder when the shoulders sag, for example, it may be necessary to take special exercises to strengthen shoulder muscles in order to protect important nerves.

I have had many cases of arm, neck, and shoulder pain that had postural connections and in which the only remedy seemed to be exercise. A middle-aged contractor, for example, who suffered from recurring muscle spasms at the base of his neck along with pain and numbness radiating down both arms into his fingers, obtained relief by doing shoulder shrugs, standing presses, and upright rowing motions (all described in this chapter) to "lift up" his shoulder girdle. (When possible, you should, of course, do barbell exercises for all of the major muscles of the body in building general, all-round body strength.)

BARBELL EXERCISES MAKE WEAK BACKS STRONG

Contrary to popular belief, you do not have to be strong to exercise with a barbell, and you do not necessarily have to increase the weight of the barbell for building greater strength. You can use light weights in all of your exercises in order to maintain a certain amount of strength and muscle tone, and you can select exercises that affect certain parts of your body if you like. But since strength is easily and rapidly developed by gradually increasing the amount of weight you use, you should take advantage of your barbell exercises by adding a few extra pounds to the bar occasionally.

In many cases, patients who are unable to get out of bed because of injury can use barbells an dumbbells right in bed to strengthen weak muscles, and they will get just as much or more benefit from such exercise than if they were up doing pushups. Patients who are too weak to do even a modified pushup, for example, can exercise the same muscles by lying on their back and pressing up a light barbell. There is hardly a muscle in the body that cannot be exercised with a barbell in a convenient posture.

HOW TO MAKE A BARBELL

If you do not have a set of store-bought barbells, you can make a "barbell" by tying a sandbag to each end of a notched broom stick. As you grow stronger, you may simply increase the amount of sand in the bags. With a little imagination, you can construct an adjustable barbell of your own design.

Most commercial barbells have a thin metal sleeve that fits loosely over the bar so that the bar can rotate freely during exercises without blistering the hands. If you make a barbell with the weight fixed securely on each end of the bar, you should slide the bar through a shorter, larger pipe to make a rotating sleeve (*before* you secure the weight to each end of the bar)—or you may simply wear gloves during your exercises. When you are using adjustable discs that rotate on the bar, you might be able to get by without the sleeve or the gloves.

Drop by your local sporting goods store and inquire about a barbell. If you do buy a barbell, make sure that you get a couple of large plates to form the basic weight of the barbell, along with a sufficient quantity of smaller plates to permit the progressive addition of a few pounds at a time as you grow stronger. Most barbell sets will already be made up of graduated plates, however, so any commercial set will probably be adequate.

To begin with, you will use about 50 pounds (including the weight of the bar, which is usually about 20 pounds) in most of your exercises, but if you are a man your strength will increase so rapidly that you will soon be using 100 pounds or more in some of your exercises. For this reason, it might be more economical to buy a heavier set (for example, 110 pounds) to begin with than to buy extra plates as you grow stronger.

Basic Rules of Progressive Resistance Exercise

Although progressive resistance exercise is relatively simple, it must be performed according to certain basic rules to be effective. There is a great deal of difference between scientific resistance exercise and haphazard calisthenics or feats of strength. Here are the questions you would ask, and the rules you should go by:

How Many Repetitions Should You Do In Each Exercise, and How Much Weight Should You Use?

RULE 1: In each exercise you do, *select a weight that can be used properly for the recommended number of repetitions,* which will be about eight in most exercises. Men should try about 50 pounds (including the weight of the bar) and women should try about 25 pounds (or use only the bar); both may then adjust the weight as necessary. For the first few weeks, of course, you should use a very light weight in order to avoid excessive muscle soreness.

After you have been using the same weight for several days, you will find it easier to do a greater number of repetitions.

How Many Sets of Each Exercise Should You Do?

RULE 2: Those beginning barbell exercises for the first time should *do only one set of each exercise in each workout for the first four weeks;* for example, if the exercise calls for eight repetitions, it should be performed eight times consecutively, and that is all.

How Often Should You Work Out?

RULE 3: Both experience and research have shown that *you can get stronger and more muscular by exercising every other day than by exercising every day*. The reason for this, of course, is that by alternating rest days and exercise days your muscles have more time to repair and rebuild in preparation for the next workout; and if you are taking progressive resistance exercise, each time the muscle fibers rebuild they get a little thicker and a little stronger.

Most persons prefer to workout on Monday, Wednesday, and Friday so that the weekend will be free for rest and recreation. In each workout, do only the amount of exercise recommended and no more! And make sure that you get all the sleep you need each night.

How Fast Should You Work Out?

RULE 4: Many people who take regular exercise believe that the faster you exercise the better. This might be the case in some types of exercise, but it certainly does not apply in the case of progressive resistance exercise. In fact, if you do not *pause between repetitions and rest a few minutes between sets,* continuous muscular contraction against resistance may obstruct the blood circulation to such an extent that you will tire prematurely and get less benefit from your exercise.

Perform each exercise through a full range of movement at a moderate rate of speed, and then pause momentarily between repetitions (at the starting point) so that muscular relaxation will permit the circulation of blood through the muscle.

Rest at least 2 minutes between sets of an exercise so that the blood circulation will have time to remove waste products (lactic acid) and replenish energy stores (glycogen).

If a particularly heavy exercise leaves you breathing heavily, continue your rest until you feel sufficiently recovered to begin another set of exercise.

What Should You Wear During Your Exercise?

RULE 5: We all know that a good workout depends upon warming up and then staying warm. This is why athletes sometimes wear shoes, socks, and sweat clothes during exercise periods. The exercise you will be taking—if you are using this book as a guide —will not be so strenuous that you will be perspiring a great deal, but *you should always be adequately clothed to prevent cooling of the skin by drafts.*

Your feet should always be covered—at least with socks—during your workout. When the feet are chilled, the whole body is affected.

What Should You Eat?

RULE 6: There is no magic formula for eating that will build muscles, but a diet that is rich in protein is important if you are to get full benefit from your exercise. Eggs, meat, fish, poultry, milk, cheese, nuts, and legumes are good protein foods. Of course, you should always have a good, all-round diet, but you should *eat a larger amount of protein foods when you are taking progressive resistance exercise.*

Try to take your exercise before eating (preferably in the evening), or at least 2 hours after eating.

Which Exercises Should You Do?

RULE 7: Even though you may be taking these exercises only to strengthen your back, it is important that you also develop supporting and overlapping muscles that aid the action of the back muscles, as I explained earlier. And you should try to make sure that all of the major muscles of the body are evenly developed so that a balanced musculature will prevent the development of abnormal stresses and strains on the spine. For this reason, *you should try to do all of the exercises described* in this chapter (that is, of course, if you are not following the exercises in Chapter 12)—if not all in one workout, then by alternating them from one workout to another. If you do not want to do all of the exercises in this chapter, you should at least do exercises 2, 4, 7, and 8, since these are the most important and the most basic for strengthening the back.

What About Breathing?

RULE 8: The rules of breathing are the same for barbell exercises as for other forms of exercise (see "How to Breathe During Your Exercises" in Chapter 12). When you are using a barbell, however, it is even more important that you do not hold your breath during your exercises.

Breathing actually aids the flow of venous blood in completing its uphill journey from the lower part of the body back to the heart. When we take a deep breath, for example, the negative pressure created by the expanding chest exerts a suction effect on the upper portion of the large vein leading back to the heart, and the downward movement of the diaphragm gives the column of blood a push from the bottom. Thus, the push-pull effect of breathing acts as a subsidiary pump in aiding the circulation of blood.

When you hold your breath during an exercise, your circulation slows down at a time when you need an *increase* in circulation. And if you take a deep breath and hold it during a heavy barbell exercise, the positive pressure in the lungs (created by the contraction of chest and abdominal muscles) might obstruct the circulation of blood enough to cause a blackout. (If you follow the instructions accompanying each exercise, you will not be making such a heavy effort, but there may be some who will be tempted to test their strength with a barbell.)

When breathing instructions do not accompany the description of any of the barbell exercises to follow, try to breathe "out" during exertion, and "in" between repetitions; otherwise, just try to breathe rhythmically and comfortably.

Gripping the Bar and Placing Your Feet

There are two ways to grip a barbell. One way is to grip the bar with your hands under the bar in a palms-up or underhand position, and another way is to grip the bar with your hands over the bar in a palms-down or overhand position. *Only the overhand grip will be used in the exercises described in this chapter.*

In all of the exercises in which you must stand, place your feet in a comfortable stance with your heels several inches apart and your toes slightly slanted out to each side.

Basic Barbell Exercises for Building Back Strength

(1) A Warmup Exercise

You already know the importance of warming up for your exercises; and once you are advanced enough to do two sets of each exercise, you can warmup for the various exercises by using a lighter weight in the first set. But to begin with, you will have to precede your workout with a good, all-round warmup exercise that will affect all of the major muscle groups. Here is such an exercise:

Stand close to a barbell so that your toes are under the bar. Squat down and grasp the bar with your hands palms down (overhand grip), shoulder-width apart. Keep both feet flat on the floor and keep your back fairly flat. In one continuous, smooth motion, lift the barbell straight up from the floor to overhead and back again. Use a light weight in this exercise and lift the bar overhead about ten times.

If you squat low with your back as vertical and as nearly flat as comfort will permit in beginning the exercise, your lower back, hips, and thighs will do most of the work until the bar is about halfway up, at which point your arms, shoulders, and upper back will complete the exercise in lifting the bar overhead.

Breathe any way you like as long as you breathe rhythmically (See Figure 33).

(2) The Standing Press *

---

* Important basic exercise.

The standing press with a barbell builds important arm, back, and shoulder muscles. And if you do this exercise correctly, you will strengthen many of the muscles responsible for keeping the shoulders square and the spine erect.

Standing erect with a barbell supported at shoulder level, press the bar overhead 8 to 10 times. Keep your back and legs straight, and look straight ahead during the exercise. You may vary the width of your grip on the bar for comfort, but you should always grip the bar with your palms facing away from you in an overhand position.

Breathe "in" while the weight is being supported at shoulder level, and then breathe "out" while the weight is being pressed overhead (See Figure 34).

(3) The Bench Press

This exercise will develop muscles on the front of your chest and shoulders, thus aiding posture by building support for your

Figure 33:   A warmup exercise (1)

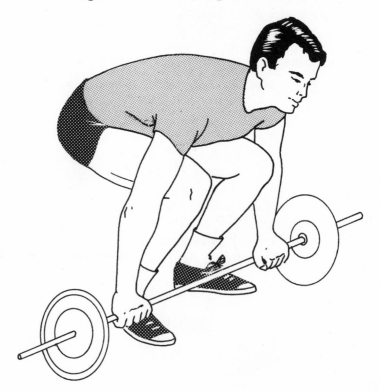

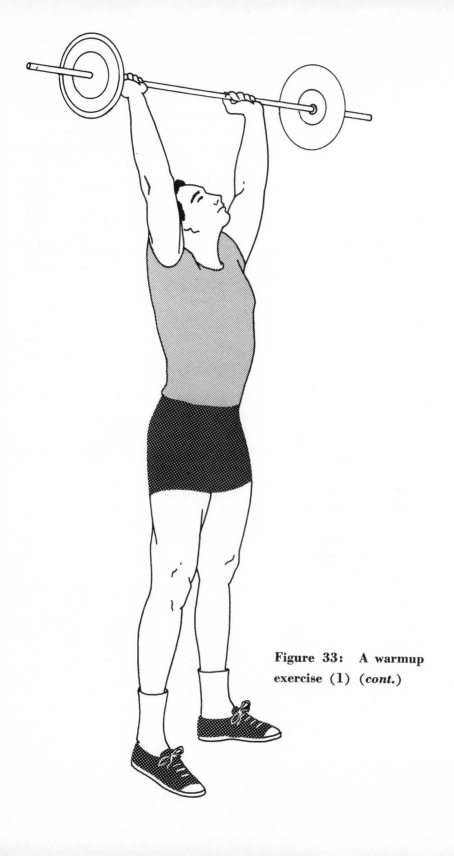

Figure 33: A warmup
exercise (1) (*cont.*)

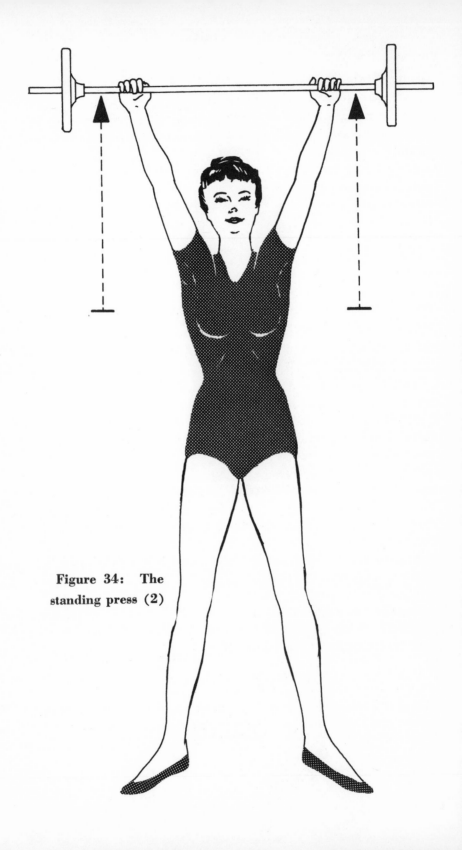

Figure 34: The standing press (2)

rib cage. Furthermore, balanced muscular development that includes the large chest muscles will support the action of back muscles in many types of work in which you must do a great deal of pushing and pulling, thus lessening the chances of back strain.

Lie on your back on a narrow padded bench (or on the floor if you do not have a bench) and press a barbell from your chest to arm's length (straight-up toward the ceiling) 8 to 10 times. Grasp the bar with an overhand grip with your hands slightly wider than shoulder-width apart.

Inhale while the weight is resting on your chest, and exhale while the weight is being pressed up.

When you begin to use a fairly heavy weight in this exercise, make sure that someone is standing by to help you place and remove the barbell from your chest (See Figure 35).

(4) The Upright Rowing Motion *

This is one of the finest exercises you can do for developing the muscles responsible for supporting the shoulder girdle.

Stand erect with a barbell supported down at arm's length in front, hands together (about one hand-width apart) with a palms-down grip, and lift the bar up under your chin. Keep your elbows pointed forward and up as you lift the bar so that the muscles in your upper back and shoulders will be forced to do most of the work. Keep your back and legs straight during this exercise. If you have to bend your knees or jerk the weight up, the barbell is too heavy.

Breathe anyway you like as long as you breathe rhythmically. Most persons prefer to breathe "in" as the weight comes up, and "out" as the weight goes down.

Upright rowing motions are especially valuable for persons who must sit around all day with their shoulders slumped over a desk or a machine (See Figure 36).

(5) The Bent-Over Rowing Motion

If you do a lot of hoeing in a garden, or if you row a boat or scrape paint off the wall of a building, you will use the same

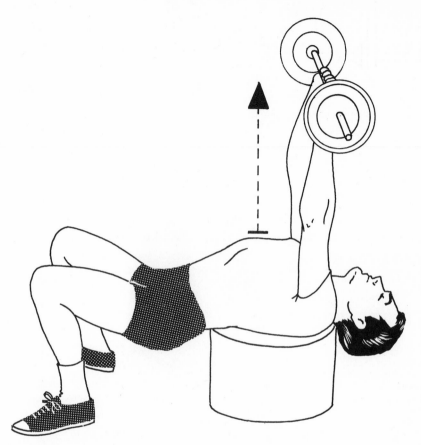

Figure 35:   The bench press (3)

muscles this exercise is designed to develop; but labor is not a substitute for exercise that results in full and even development of a muscle through a complete range of movement. Properly performed exercises, however, will improve your ability to work, as well as provide additional protection against strain during exertion.

Bent-over rowing motions are designed to strengthen upper back muscles that pull the arms down and back, but the position in which the exercise is performed also provides a considerable amount of exercise for the lower back.

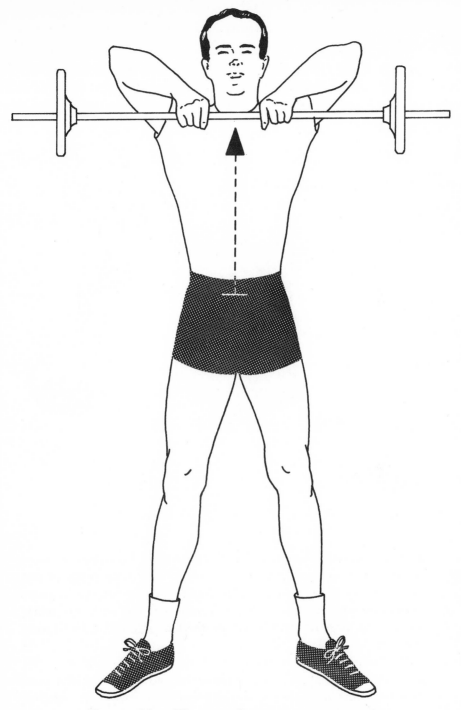

Figure 36: The upright rowing motion (4)

Bend over from your hips with your back flat and your knees bent and grasp a barbell with an overhand grip, hands slightly wider than shoulder-width apart. Lift the barbell from the floor to your beltline. Keep your elbows close to your sides—and do not jerk the weight up (See Figure 37).

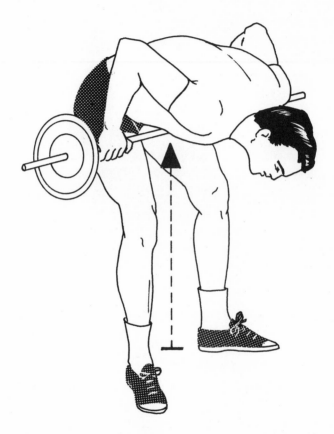

Figure 37: The bent-over rowing motion (5)

It is important to keep your back flat during this exercise, but you may bend your knees as necessary. Do not use so much weight that you cannot do about eight repetitions without straining or cheating. If you have a history of recurring low-back trouble, leave this exercise off your list and do the chinning exercises described in Group 8 of Chapter 12.

In bent-over rowing motions, you should inhale when you lower the barbell, and exhale when you lift the barbell.

(6) The Good Morning Exercise

This exercise is designed to strengthen low-back and hip muscles and to stretch tight muscles and tendons up and down the back of your legs. You know from reading other portions of this book that short hamstrings can cause backache, so you should include an exercise that will stretch these structures forcefully but safely.

Stand erect with a light barbell supported across your shoulders behind your neck. Keeping your back flat and your legs straight, bend forward by bending at the hips only. Stop the bending the moment you begin to feel uncomfortable. As you become more flexible and more accustomed to the exercise, however, you should be able to bend farther forward without any discomfort. Do the exercise six to eight times (See Figure 38).

Obviously, you must use a very light weight in this exercise if you want to avoid strain. Begin by using only the bar, and then gradually add a few pounds as comfort permits.

The technique used in performing this "good morning exercise" must *never* be used in supporting heavy weights or in lifting objects from the floor! *Do not do this exercise if you have back trouble!*

Exhale while bending over, and inhale while returning to an erect position.

(7) The Bent-Knee Dead Lift *

Of all the exercises that will improve your ability to lift heavy objects correctly and safely, the bent-knee dead lift with a barbell is perhaps the best. The technique used in this lift duplicates good lifting technique, and it will develop muscles in the thighs, hips, and low back that are most important in "lifting with your legs."

Stand close to a barbell so that your toes are under the bar. Squat down with your back flat and your hips low and grasp the bar with an overhand grip. Keep both feet parallel and flat on the floor in a comfortable stance. Using only your legs and hips, stand erect with the barbell so that you are supporting the weight

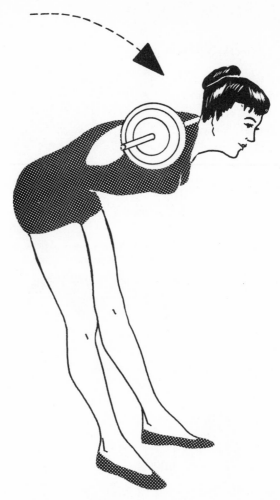

Figure 38: The good morning exercise (6)

in a dead hang down at arm's length in front. It will, of course,
be necessary to tilt your upper body forward when beginning
the lift, but if you will keep your back fairly flat there will not
be any dangerous strain on your spine (see Figure 39).

  You will be able to work up to a fairly heavy weight in this
exercise, but you should be slow and cautious in your progress.
Do not use so much weight that you have to strain in completing
eight repetitions.

Breathe anyway you like as long as you do not hold your breath.

(8) The Flat-Footed Squat *

Squatting with both feet flat on the floor is also a good low-back, hip, and thigh exercise, and it is a key exercise in acquiring the strength and ability needed to use correct lifting techniques.

With a barbell supported across your shoulders behind your neck, squat down until the back of your thighs begin to press against your calves and then come back up. Keep your back flat and both feet flat on the floor. If you have short ankle tendons

Figure 39: The bent-knee dead lift (7)

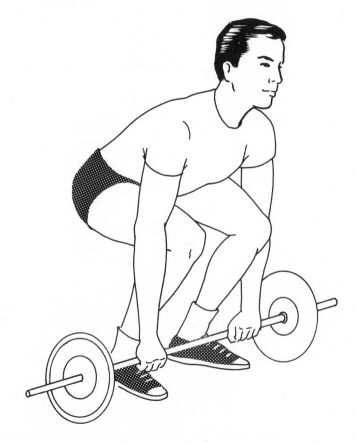

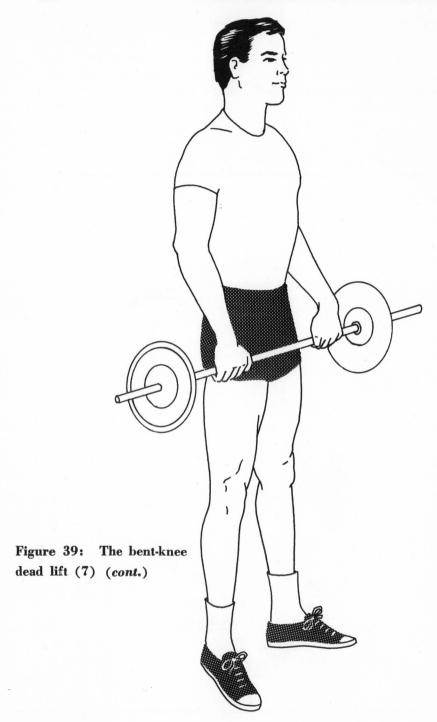

Figure 39: **The bent-knee dead lift (7) (*cont.*)**

you may have to do your squats with a thick board under your heels to begin with, but with a little practice you should eventually be able to squat flat-footed. In order to squat flat-footed, you will have to let your trunk tilt forward slightly, so make sure that you keep your back flat (see Figure 40).

Figure 40:   The flat-footed squat (8)

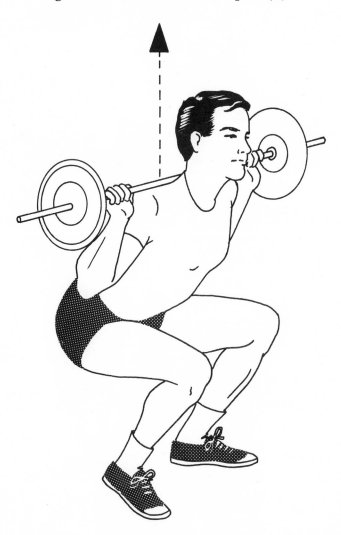

This is another exercise in which you may eventually work up to using fairly heavy weights, so it would be a good idea to have a training partner who can help you remove the weight from your shoulders if you should "over-do it" on occasions. Many gyms have "squat racks" which support the barbell at shoulder level so that you can lift the bar onto and off of your shoulders by backing up to the rack.

Do not hold your breath during squatting exercises! Breathe "in" while you are in the erect standing position, and then breathe "out" during the actual squat. (See Rule 8 in this chapter.)

(9) The Stiff-Arm Pullover

This exercise was described in Chapter 12 for use with a sand-bag. But since you are using barbells in the exercises in this chapter, the stiff-arm pullover can be performed more effectively in the following manner:

Lie on your back on a padded bench (or on the floor) with your head near the end of the bench. Holding a barbell at arm's length over your chest (using an overhand grip with your hands about shoulder-width apart), let the barbell down and back over your head with slightly bent elbows. *Inhale deeply as the weight goes back.* You should use a very light weight in this exercise if you want to force full expansion of your chest. When the weight is too heavy, excessive muscular contraction will keep the ribs from spreading apart (see Figure 41).

If you will do your stiff-arm pullovers immediately after your squatting exercises, you can take full advantage of the breathlessness resulting from the squats in stretching your rib cage. (All of the exercises in this chapter are arranged in a certain order so that each exercise will prepare you for the exercise to follow. So try to do them in the order suggested.)

A deep, flexible, and well-supported rib cage is important in maintaining a straight spine, and the exercises designed to expand your chest will take the hump out of your back and the pot out of your belly.

(10) Toe Rises With a Barbell

Group 9 in Chapter 12 contains descriptions of a couple of exercises that are designed to stretch backache-causing short

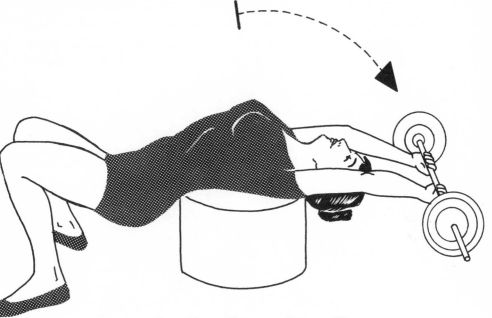

Figure 41:   The stiff-arm pullover (9)

ankle tendons, but none of these are quite as effective as barbell toe rises from a thick board. The reason for this, of course, is that the additional weight of the barbell across the shoulders forces the heels to drop lower than with bodyweight alone; and the increased resistance offers a much more effective stimulus for development of the calf muscles.

With a barbell supported across your shoulders behind your neck, stand on a thick board (for example, a 2x4) with your weight supported on the front part of your feet. Rise up and down on your toes 15 to 20 times, letting your heels drop as low as possible. In order to avoid a painful reaction in your calves from the stretching of short muscles, however, you should do only a few repetitions with bodyweight alone for several days before using a barbell.

Occasionally do your toe rises with your toes pointed inward, that is, in a pigeon-toed manner, so that you will strengthen the muscles supporting the arch of your foot (see Figure 42).

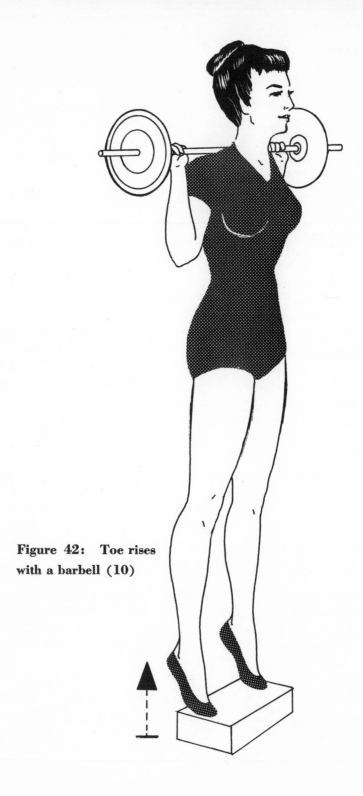

Figure 42: Toe rises
with a barbell (10)

(11) Situps and Leg Raises *

Although some of the barbell exercises will provide a certain amount of exercise for your abdominal muscles, you should include an abdominal exercise in order to make sure that your muscular development is balanced for maximum support of your spine.

Turn to Group 3 in Chapter 12 for instructions in performing abdominal exercises.

(12) Maintaining Flexibility

Contrary to the once popular belief that barbell exercises will make you stiff and "muscle-bound," it is now well known that such exercise results in an *increase* in flexibility and in speed of movement. No other form of exercise utilizes such a full range of joint movement with full extension and contraction of the muscles as scientific barbell and dumbbell exercises, and there is hardly a school or college in the nation that does not recommend the use of weights for improving athletic ability. So you can forget the old muscle-bound myth that so many people once associated with using barbells.

Since none of the barbell exercises described in this chapter call for any side-bending or rotary movements, you might want to include some of the bending and twisting exercises described in Group 1 of Chapter 12 for maximum spinal flexibility. You might also want to take the thigh-band-flexibility exercise in Group 10 if the test accompanying the exercise gives you a positive sign.

Summary

1. Since there are a fairly large number of exercises described in this chapter, you may not want to do all of them in one workout. If not, just alternate them in different workouts until you cover all of them—or select the exercises you feel you need to do.
2. Remember that these barbell exercises build muscular strength for your back that can be put to practical use in everyday activities, and they will improve your posture as well as your muscle guard. Anyone can take barbell exercises.

Basic Rules In a Nutshell

- In selecting a weight to use in an exercise, always pick a weight that you can use several times without strain.
- After a couple of weeks of performing very light exercises, add enough weight to the bar to tax your strength within the recommended number of repetitions.
- As you become stronger and you are able to easily exceed the recommended number of repetitions, add enough weight to the bar to keep the exercise moderately resistant.
- After about four weeks of training, do two sets of each exercise if you like, using the first set as a light warmup for a heavier weight in the second set.
- Try to schedule your workouts every other day. You can make better progress by alternating rest days with workout days.
- Perform each exercise through a full range of movement, and then pause between repetitions and rest a few minutes between sets.
- Make sure that you are adequately clothed during your workouts if there are drafts of cool air in your training area.
- Do not hold your breath during barbell exercises!

14

Questions and Answers on What You Learned in This Book About Your Back

If you want to keep active and productive as the years roll by, you will have to take care of your back just as you would a piece of machinery or a fruit tree. And if you do observe all of the rules of good posture, exercise, and other self-help measures outlined in this book, your general health will benefit immeasurably. So you have nothing to lose and everything to gain by adopting a preventive program of back care that you can follow every day of your life.

By putting into effect what you learn from reading this book, your back will be stronger for a more productive life, and you will feel better for a longer, happier life.

225

A Backache Guide for Laymen

Backache—Home Treatment and Prevention is a book you will want to read again and again in preventing the development of backache, and you will be referring to it frequently in taking care of your back problems as they arise; so keep it on the shelf, and try to see to it that it is read by every member of the family. If you are an employer, recommend this book to your employees; the benefit they will obtain from reading it will reflect itself in increased production and in decreased medical expenses.

How Much Do You Know About Your Back?

If you have already read this book completely, test your "back knowledge" with this true or false quiz. The answers, with explanations, can be found on pages 229-232.

	True	*False*
1. The cervical spine is the same as the neck.	___	___
2. The coccyx is at the bottom of the spine.	___	___
3. Situps are better for the abdomen and easier on the back if they are performed with the knees bent.	___	___
4. Correct lifting means keeping your legs straight and lifting with your back.		
5. When your posture is perfect, there are no visible curves in your spine.	___	___
6. You have 26 vertebrae and 23 discs.	___	___
7. When you sit, there should be a slight arch in your lower back.	___	___
8. Some doctors can cure arthritis.	___	___
9. Sciatica is an infection caused by raw pork.	___	___
10. Dry heat is better than moist heat.	___	___
11. Torn muscles are best treated with cold packs for the first 24 to 48 hours.	___	___
12. It is better to sleep on your stomach than to sleep on your back.	___	___
13. You should never put a pillow under your knees when you are lying on your back.	___	___

True   *False*

14. If you exercise with barbells, you can get stronger by working out every day than by working out every other day.   ____   ____

15. A person with a suspected broken neck should be transported face down.   ____   ____

16. Traction is used to relieve pressure on spinal nerves.   ____   ____

17. Muscle spasm is a common cause of neck "cricks."   ____   ____

18. Spinal curvatures cannot be detected in children.   ____   ____

19. Sixteen years of age is soon enough to begin correcting a spinal curvature.   ____   ____

20. If you suddenly develop a "hump" in your back, it means that you have a vertebra out of place.   ____   ____

21. If you develop acute back pain with fever, you should wait until the fever subsides before seeing a doctor.   ____   ____

22. Weak muscles and poor posture are not a common cause of backache.   ____   ____

23. A spinal curvature that an adult has had all his life can be corrected by manipulation.   ____   ____

24. There are seven vertebrae in the lumbar portion of your spine.   ____   ____

25. The lumbosacral joints are the most common site of back trouble.   ____   ____

26. A "slipped disc" always requires surgery.   ____   ____

27. It is possible for back trouble to cause arm or leg pain.   ____   ____

28. When you have back pain, there is always something wrong with your back.   ____   ____

29. When you sit up in bed, you should keep your legs flat on the mattress.   ____   ____

30. It is possible to get an infection in your vertebrae by drinking unpasteurized milk.   ____   ____

	True	*False*
31. Women who have worn high-heeled shoes for many years should switch to shoes with no heels at all.	____	____
32. Spina bifida is a cleft spine.	____	____
33. Exposure to cold is a common cause of muscle spasm.	____	____
34. One of the most important aspects of good posture is a flat abdomen.	____	____
35. You should take a deep breath and hold it when you are doing an exercise.	____	____
36. If you cannot touch your toes with your legs straight, you should use momentum in your toe-touching exercises.	____	____
37. Strong abdominal muscles are just as important as strong back muscles in keeping the spine straight.	____	____
38. The condition of your feet and shoes has nothing to do with back trouble.	____	____
39. Fat people never have a backache.	____	____
40. It is better to sleep directly on a board than to put it between the mattress and the springs.	____	____
41. Your automobile seat should be moved back so that your leg is straight when your foot is on the gas pedal.	____	____
42. When you are carrying a heavy object, you should always let it rest against your body.	____	____
43. You can "slip a disc" by sneezing while you are bent over.	____	____
44. When you are pushing your car, you should keep your spine in line with the driving force of your legs.	____	____
45. Prolonged nervous tension can cause a backache.	____	____
46. A head piece installed on the back of an automobile seat is designed to prevent whiplash injuries.	____	____

	True	*False*
47. Crippling rheumatoid arthritis rarely occurs before 50 years of age.	———	———
48. Exercise helps to prevent osteoporosis in old people.	———	———
49. Once your doctor prescribes a back support, you should wear it permanently.	———	———
50. If you have a backache caused by sitting or standing all day, exercise might be effective in relieving your symptoms.	———	———

Answers and Explanations for Quiz

Subtract two points for each incorrect answer. A score of 86 or higher is good; 74 to 84, fair; and below 72, poor.

1. *True.* From top to bottom, there are 5 main sections in the spine: cervical, dorsal, lumbar, sacral, and coccygeal.
2. *True.* The coccyx is also known as the "tail bone."
3. *True.* Bending the knees in situps lessens leverage on the lumbar spine, making it easier to exercise the abdominal muscles.
4. *False.* In correct lifting technique, you should keep your back flat, squat low, and then lift with your legs.
5. *False.* The spine should appear to be straight when viewed from the back, but when viewed from the side the normal curves of the spine should be visible.
6. *True.* There is no disc or cushion between the skull and the first vertebra, between the first and second vertebrae, or between the sacrum and the coccyx.
7. *True.* You should try to maintain the normal lumbar curve when sitting.
8. *False.* There is no known cure for arthritis at the present time—although the disease can be controlled, or symptoms can be relieved, with proper treatment.
9. *False.* Sciatica is a nerve pain radiating down into the leg.
10. *False.* Moist heat is more effective than dry heat.
11. *True.* Cold packs applied to a fresh injury will cut down on bleeding and swelling.

12. *False.* The normal curves of the spine are best maintained by sleeping on your back.

13. *False.* A pillow under both knees will very often relieve backache by relieving stress on the lumbar spine. However, persons with spinal rheumatoid arthritis should *not* use a pillow under their knees!

14. *False.* Every-other-day training with barbells builds greater strength by allowing time for recovery.

15. *False.* A person with a broken neck should be placed face up, while a person with a broken back should be placed face down.

16. *True.* Traction pulls the vertebrae apart to widen the openings through which the spinal nerves pass.

17. *True.* Most "cricks" are caused by muscle spasm that will usually go away in three or four days.

18. *False.* Every child under 13 years of age should be examined regularly for spinal curvature.

19. *False.* Most spinal curvatures must be corrected before the child reaches 12 years of age if full correction is to be made—although treatment should be continued until he reaches 16 years of age.

20. *False.* A sudden development of a "hump" in your back may be an indication of a fracture or a bone disease. See your doctor.

21. *False.* Backache accompanied by a fever is usually indicative of infection, which should be treated immediately.

22. *False.* Weak muscles and poor posture, along with incorrect lifting techniques, are the most common causes of backache.

23. *False.* A curvature of long standing in an adult is structural in nature and cannot be fully corrected.

24. *False.* There are only five vertebrae in the lumbar spine.

25. *True.* Most back trouble occurs in the lumbosacral joints at the bottom of the spine where weight bearing is greatest.

26. *False.* Orthopedic authorities tell us that about 80 percent of all slipped discs will recover under prolonged physical treatment.

27. *True.* Spinal nerves irritated in the vertebral column can refer pain into any portion of the body.

28. *False.* Many organic diseases refer pain into the structures of a normal back.

29. *False.* Always bend your knees when sitting up in bed if you want to avoid a sacroiliac strain.

30. *True.* The germs of brucellosis and tuberculosis are sometimes found in unpasteurized milk, and they actually invade the bone of the vertebrae.

31. *False.* Women who are accustomed to wearing high-heeled shoes may develop acute backache from tension over shortened hamstrings if they suddenly switch to shoes without heels.

32. *True.* Spina bifida is a birth defect in which a portion of the spine fails to close with normal bone development.

33. *True.* Chilled muscles very often become inflamed.

34. *True.* Even when the spine is straight, a fat, bulging abdomen can ruin good posture by letting the abdominal organs fall.

35. *False.* Holding your breath during an exercise might interfere with the flow of blood to your brain and cause a blackout.

36. *False.* Using force or momentum in a toe-touching exercise can strain your sacroiliac joints.

37. *True.* Muscle support on both sides of the spine is important in maintaining a strong and straight spine.

38. *False.* Many backaches are caused by bad feet and poorly fitted shoes.

39. *False.* Obesity by itself is a common cause of backache.

40. *False.* A mattress should be firm, but not so hard that it cannot mold itself to the normal curves of the spine.

41. *False.* Move your automobile seat up close enough to the gas pedal to allow your lower leg to rest at nearly a right angle to your thigh.

42. *True.* Trying to carry a heavy object without it touching your body will place a terrific amount of strain on your lower back.

43. *True.* Sneezing while bending over to tie a shoe lace or while picking up a heavy object will place a tremendous amount of pressure on the intervertebral discs.

44. *True.* You can avoid injurious leverage on your spine by keeping your back straight and in line with the driving force of your legs when you are pushing or pulling.

45. *True.* Nervous tension is a very common cause of backache.

46. *True.* Your car should have a head piece to keep your head from being snapped backward in automobile accidents.

47. *False.* Rheumatoid arthritis usually begins between the ages

of 25 and 50, whereas osteoarthritis usually makes its appearance in old age.

48. *True.* Bones are made stronger when they are placed under stress by exercise.

49. *False.* Back supports should be discarded gradually as the back becomes stronger.

50. *True.* Exercise stimulates circulation and relieves binding fatigue in muscles and joints.

Index

A

Abdomen, and posture, 139
Acute Torticollis, 68-70
"Adult rickets," 83, 84
Arthritis:
  gouty arthritis, 80
  mustard plasters, 95, 96
  osteoarthritis, 77, 78
  rheumatoid arthritis, 79, 80

B

Back:
  back trouble above the waistline, 66-72
  exercising isometrically, 198
  general disorders of, 73-85
  massage, 97-100
  most common back injury, 49, 50
  muscles located in, 38-40
  persistent back pain, 17, 18
  structural defects, 9
Backache guide for laymen, a, 226
  back trouble in disguise, 44, 45
  "back trouble" that isn't back trouble, 42-44
  caused by a short leg, 3
  common causes of, 19, 21
  correct lifting techniques, 21, 22
  diagnosis, importance of, 18, 19
  exercises for prevention and correction:
    "back-limbering" bending exercises, 174-177

Backache guide for laymen (*cont.*)
  exercises for prevention and correction (*cont.*)
    "back-straightening" exercises, 177-179
    "chest-out" breathing exercises, 185, 186
    chinning exercises, 191, 192
    developing muscles, 168-170
    five preliminary exercises, 165-168
    how to begin, 172-174
    how to breathe, 174
    incorrect exercising, case of, 4-6
    isometric exercise, 197, 198
    neck exercises, 195, 197
    progressive exercise without apparatus, 172
    pushups, 188, 190
    "shoulders-back" exercises, 186, 188
    squatting exercises, 181-185
    "stomach-in" exercises, 179-181
    stretching ankle tendons, 193
    test for tight thigh bands, 193, 195
    why you should exercise, 170
  general pattern of chronic backache, 24, 25
  home treatment, 6, 7, 86-114
  how a housewife rid herself of backache, case of, 171, 172
  in relation to posture, 2-4
  lumbosacral joints, relation to, 35
  major cause of, 48, 49
  muscle spasm, 60-64
  mustard plasters, 95, 96

233